# ENGLISH FOR NURSES

# ENGLISH FOR NURSES

**Mallika Balu** MA Eng
Lecturer
Department of English
Surana College, Bengaluru, India

***Foreword***
R Shashidhar

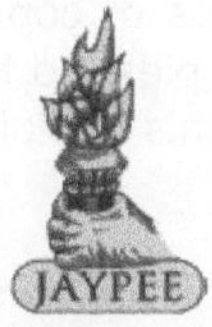


**JAYPEE BROTHERS MEDICAL PUBLISHERS (P) LTD**

**New Delhi • London**

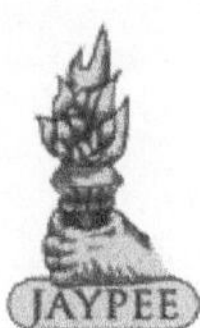

**Jaypee Brothers Medical Publishers (P) Ltd.**

**Headquarters**

EMCA House
23/23-B, Ansari Road, Daryaganj
New Delhi 110 002, India
Landline: +91-11-23272143,
+91-11-23272703+91-11-23282021,
+91-11-23245672
E-mail: jaypee@jaypeebrothers.com

**Overseas Off ce**

JP Medical Ltd.
83, Victoria Street, London
SW1H 0HW (UK)
Phone: +44-20 3170 8910
E-mail: info@jpmedpub.com

**Corporate Office**

Jaypee Brothers Medical Publishers (P) Ltd.
4838/24, Ansari Road, Daryaganj
New Delhi 110 002, India
Phone: +91-11-43574357
Fax: +91-11-43574314
E-mail: jaypee@jaypeebrothers.com

**EU GPSR** Authorised Representative

Logos Europe, 9 rue Nicolas Poussin
17000, La Rochelle, France
Phone: +33 (0) 6 67 93 73 78
E-mail: Contact@logoseurope.eu

Website: www.jaypeebrothers.com
Website: www.jaypeedigital.com



***English for Nurses***

*First Edition:* 2011

*Reprint:* **2025**

ISBN: 978-93-5025-100-3

Printed in India

*To*

*Late Prof Sham Iyengar*
*who was my mentor*
*in the Open Science Lab*
*and guided me in developing*
*a positive approach to research*

# Foreword

*English for Nurses* begins with a historical perspective of the English language and gradually moves onto delineate its evolution, over the centuries, into the present non-native English. Subtly, but gradually, the author refers to the way it has acquired the status of a global language and the need for learning it as an important tool to communicate not only in our day-to-day transactions but also for communicating in professional contexts. One of the salient aspects of the book is providing the landscape of language to the text, before the author ventures into her main concern.

The first part of the book treks through challenging terrains of English Grammar with consummate ease and it familiarises the users to these aspects of Grammar in the context of the special purpose that the book addresses at the world level.

The second part deals with 'Sentence' and its varieties. The third part aims at developing other major language learning skills—particularly Reading and Writing . The various chapters in the book are meaningfully integrated with the field of nursing and medicine. Every item of Grammar introduced and illustrated is accompanied by exercises and tasks, which are meant to reinforce learning.

These exercises are drawn abundantly from the field of nursing and medicine besides from day-to-day life situations, which makes the text highly comprehensive. This synthesis of the professional and real-life situations makes the acquisition of the target language "immediate" to the learner. Quite often, the author takes pain to go into the etymology of certain terms to avoid the mechanical use of the terms by learners. This is a very rare quality in a book of the nature.

The minuteness of details that the author provides wherever necessary, the fluid movement from one stage to another in the text, the lucidity of style and clarity of thought make the book user-friendly and fulfill the need of the hour.

I will not be surprised if this well-researched, highly organized, meticulously written *English for Nurses* compels a place for itself in academic libraries, all over.

**R Shashidhar**
Faculty
Regional Institute of English, South India
Jhanabharathi Campus
Bengaluru, India

# Preface

To write any book involves insightful hard work. But, if the book in question happens to be a book on Grammar, it is challenging. So has it been the writing of this book *English for Nurses.* When I accepted to write this book, I faced two major facts. One, I had to incorporate the wonderful healing world of a student nurse. Two, it is very different from teaching Literature and General English as I have been doing all these years. The ordinary college world of fun-loving teenagers is far removed from the interesting, dedicated and scientific terminology wielding world of the nursing staff. It was interesting to do this project as I learnt a lot.

Any student nurse belonging to a non-English-speaking country faces a terrible ordeal in not knowing the English language. Added to this confusion, there are new subjects both in theory and practicals to cope up with. The many techniques that have been incorporated in my classes have had the chance to be included here. The basic information on the English language, the breakdown of various topics and a detailed explanation wherever necessary have been given. This kind of explanation is vital to remove any form of doubts students get while learning a new language. At the same time, all this makes the student more interested in doing the necessary exercises. At the end or in the middle of a chapter, a chart has been provided. This helps in easy recall of the topics at hand. It also helps the students in being informed about different methods they can learn to remember and recall the information they are taking in. The repetitive reminders about a certain Grammar point helps in correct learning.

A student nurse encounters multiple worlds. One world is that of learning, the other world is that of emotionally growing into a responsible and mature adult and yet another world, that of communication. In the present age, this third world is the most unpredictable one as international boundaries have receded in people interaction. Here the knowledge of science, medicine and language has to be mixed well with the empathy and firmness in dealing with live situations. This book has been designed to help in dealing with this world of communication. A mixture of the scientific world as well as the general life outside the hospital is given while learning English in this book. Learning any language, more so English, is not limited to just one world (classroom and textbooks) of a student nurse. Thus, the general life—going to a movie, shopping, etc. are also featured here to help you in using your new found knowledge.

This book has been divided into parts. Each part helps the learner to attain confidence by learning in a methodical manner. Every aspect of Grammar is important in language learning. Skipping any one may lead to confusion or wrong usage by the learner. The passages given in this book throw insight into various aspects of life and when read aloud, these passages help in improving pronunciation.

The teachers may use all the exercises as given here or lessen them in class as the demands of time are met. But writing all the exercises helps a learner to become well-versed in the target language.

I sincerely hope that you will enjoy learning English in a painless way. I do stress that practice makes a learner perfect. So leave no exercise incomplete; and read, write and speak English as much as you can.

Wish you all the best.

**Mallika Balu**

# Acknowledgements

A project of this magnitude requires a lot of people interaction. When I went ahead with the task at hand, various people contributed for its success. I take this opportunity to thank them all.

My mother, Smt Kamala MS Balu, has been a pillar of strength throughout. Many were the times, I took her help in knowing whether details sounded right. She helped in typing quite a few chapters as well. My father for taking care of my pet as I was busy reading, writing and meeting people for this project.

My students Preetam, Vedavrata, Sudeep, Sushma, Supreeta of final year BA (OE); Brinda from II year BA (OE) Priya and Preeti from final year BCom, NS Toushit from II year BBM for typing many chapters and giving vital inputs by reminding me of many techniques I had used in class which I have incorporated here.

My colleague Rakshith for the grammar discussions we had, without which I could have gone into too unwanted details.

Dr Jayakumar, Prof and Head, Department of Neuro-Radiology, Senior Consultant, Khoula Hospital, Muscat, for all the technical information and corrections.

Dr Suresh for clearing the little doubts I had and sharing a few anecdotes that are here.

Smt Gowri MS for giving me first-hand information of the nursing students who struggle with English.

My friend Savitha BG helped me in typing four main chapters and Savitha GV for typing the first chapter.

Mr Srinivas, HOD , Ravi Havanur, Sathya Sujay Kumar and Ravi Shankar of the Computer Department in Surana College where help was given whenever I asked for.

Prof Manu Chakravarthi for encouraging me and directing me to Dr R Shashidhar.

Dr R Shashidhar for reading through the entire work and agreeing to write the Foreword .

Last but not least, M/s Jaypee Brothers Medical Publishers (P) Ltd, for entrusting me with such a challenging project and opening my horizons to another profession that is very different from the teaching profession I am in. All the staff there with whom I have interacted for this project.

I thank all of them for the pleasant time I had in completing this project.

# Acknowledgments

A project of this magnitude requires a lot of people interaction. When I was entrusted with the task of writing, [illegible] people contributed for its success. I take this opportunity to thank them all.

[illegible]

# Contents

## Part I

**Part II**



**Part III**

# Contents

## Part IV



## Part V

# Part I

- Brief Introduction to English
- The Sentence
- Parts of Speech
- All About Nouns
- All About Adjectives
- All About Pronouns
- All About Verbs
- All About Adverbs
- All About Prepositions
- All About Conjunctions
- All About Interjections
- Question Forms

Chapter 1

# Brief Introduction to English

A language is the speech of people. The history of a language is, therefore, the history of people. English is part of the Indo-European family of languages. The diagram shows how English came about.

## Indo-European

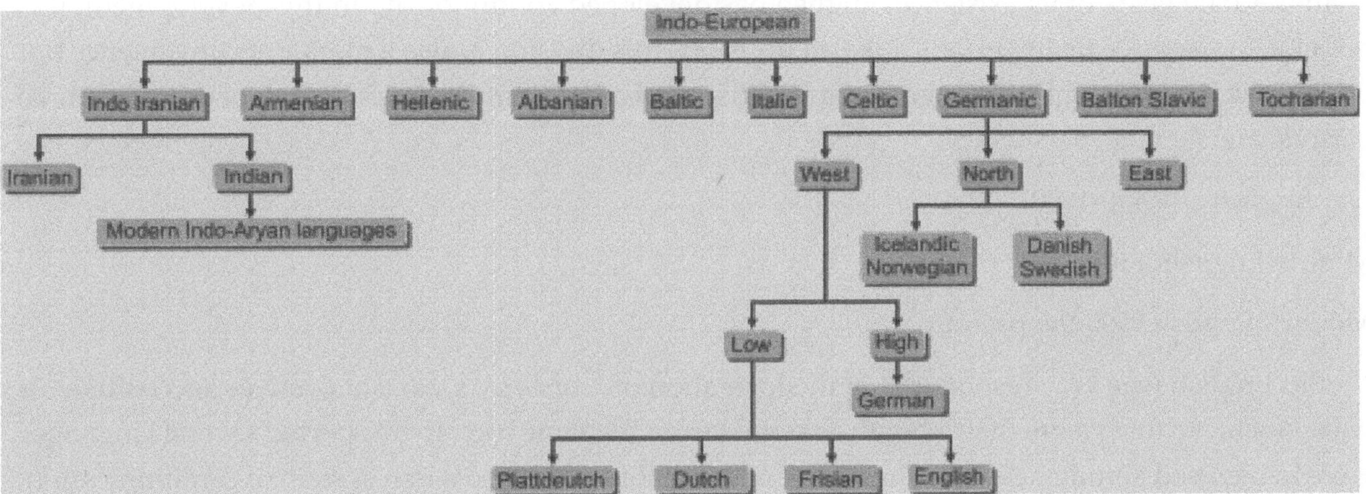


The diagram shows only lines of descent. The diagram shows the sub-branches of only the Germanic branch and the place of English in this sub-family.

Modern English belongs to the Germanic group of Indo-European languages. In the history of making of English, some movements and events stand out: 5th and 6th century migration of the three Germanic tribes: Jutes, Saxons and Angles to what is now known as England; St. Augustine's arrival in 597 and the conversion of England to Latin Christianity; 8th, 9th, and 10th century

Scandinavian invasions; the Norman conquest in the 11th century; the revival of learning in the 16th century; the settlement of North America, Australia and South Africa by the English-speaking people in the 19th century and the political colonization of India and others in the same century.

The name 'English' means 'the speech of the Anglii,' the Angles, one of the three related tribes that settled in Britannia beginning 5th century—then from Jutland came the first tribe and settled in Kent and Southern Hampshire; Saxons from Holstein next settled south of the Thames; the Angles from Schleswig settled last north of the Thames. The Germanic name of the Angles was *Angli* which became *Engle* in Old English. After 1000 AD *Englaland* was used to denote the Germanic peoples in Britain—the language was always known as *Englise.*

In the next five hundred years or so it developed into an independent language that stood out from any Germanic language spoken in Europe. It has been claimed that of all the tongues descended from Indo-European, "English has had most contacts with its kindred near and far".



In the 1500 years of its existence, English has developed continuously. In this development, it is possible to see three main periods. Like all divisions this division is also a matter of convenience but one in which it is possible to recognise certain distinguishing characteristics in each period. The three periods are:

Old English 450-1100

Middle English 1100-1500

Modern English 1500-the present

Old English was very resourceful in the formation of words by means of prefixes and suffixes; it was possible to form more than a hundred words from the same root. In this period several languages were being used simultaneously. Their contact inevitably produced a rich system of communication.

The Middle English period is the time when changes occurred in every aspect of the language. This was due to the conquering of England by the French, known familiarly as the Norman Conquest in 1066. Later on with William the Conqueror becoming the King of England, the entire English ruling class was replaced by a French aristocracy and the French language removed English of its rightful place. A century later, with the loss of Normandy, the ruling class began to think in English and thus English was slowly revived. In 14th century Geoffrey Chaucer (1350 -1400) used English in poetry. *Canterbury Tales* is the name of the famous work. He was called the 'Father of English Poetry'. John Wycliffe, translator of the Bible, belongs to this period. 15th century saw the extended use of

English as a literary medium and had a number of respected and famous writers of prose. This age gave the language a great boost leading to the Elizabethan age and to Shakespeare in particular. With Shakespeare, English language stood on the brink of Modern Period. In the Modern English Period, Grammatically, English became an analytical language. In the hands of Shakespeare and others, English was perfected as the correct medium for both prose and poetry. Conscious efforts were made to make it the acceptable language for science; spelling reforms were undertaken. Dictionaries were composed and English was spread in other lands giving rise to new, *non-native varieties of English.*

The evolution of the word 'English' is very interesting and is in some ways symbolic of the development of the English language. The word is derived from the name of the Angles who along with the Jutes and Saxons founded settlement in England in the fifth and sixth centuries. The Angles got their name from the 'angle' or corner of the land that juts out into the Southern Baltic between the modern towns of Schleswig and Flensburg. In Latin and Germanic their name was '*Angli*' which later became '*Engle*' by a change of the stressed vowel. Before 1000AD '*Angelcynn*' (Angle-race) was used to denote collectively the Germanic people in England, the Jutes, Saxons and Angles alike. After 1000 AD *England* (Land of the Angles) became popular.

Today English language is made up of 26 letters. They are–

**A B C D E F G H I J K L M N O P Q R S T U V W X Y Z**

There are two ways of writing them; Upper case alphabets and Lower case alphabets.

**A B C D E F G H I J K L M N O P Q R S T U V W X Y Z**

**are Upper case alphabets. They are also called as Capital letters.**

**a b c d e f g h i j k l m n o p q r s t u v w x y z**

**are called as Lower case letters. They are also called as Small letters.**

These are divided into two groups–Vowels and Consonants.

**a e i o u**

**are called Vowels**

**b c d f g h j k l m n p q r s t v w x y z**

**are called Consonants**

The rules of forming words, sentences and speech are called the study of English Grammar and Linguistics. Here we learn the basic rules of English Grammar. Welcome to all the students to know and improve English.

Here is a small table to show how English spellings changed from 13th century to modern days.

| Chaucer's Spelling | Shakespeare's Spelling | Modern Spelling |
|---|---|---|
| lyf | leif | life |
| deed | di:d | deed |
| deel | de:l | deal |
| name | ne::m | name |
| hoom | ho:m | home |
| hous | hous | house |

## Importance of the English Language

Just as the history of the English language is interesting, so are the reasons for studying the English language. Any student, who takes up the task of learning English, asks the question, why should he/ she study the language? This brings us to the importance of learning English.

# Brief Introduction to English

English is the first language of the United Kingdom and a few of its former colonies like the United States of America, Canada, and Australia. In common means of communication English is used between the peoples of different nations. The UNO has given English the status of being an official language. Thus, it can be called as an international language.

These days every country needs the help of another country for various reasons. More so in the political and economic arena. English is, therefore, being learnt and used all over the world not out of any imposition but by the realization that there are advantages in learning the language. It is no longer the language of Great Britain only.

Graduate students and scholars need to consult libraries to maintain standards in education and to get higher knowledge. Good reference books are found in English especially in science subjects. Thus English plays an important role as a library language in higher education.

Finally as a tool for communication English plays an important role in the everyday life of people across the world. Communicating thoughts and feelings is a part of language. People from different languages communicate through English. This brings people closer and encourages inter-cultural togetherness.

Thus, English has emerged as a single, powerful communication tool which helps in progress. Therefore, learning English becomes imperative.

Welcome to the wonderful and interesting arena of learning English. I hope your journey with the language is filled with interesting and happy moments.

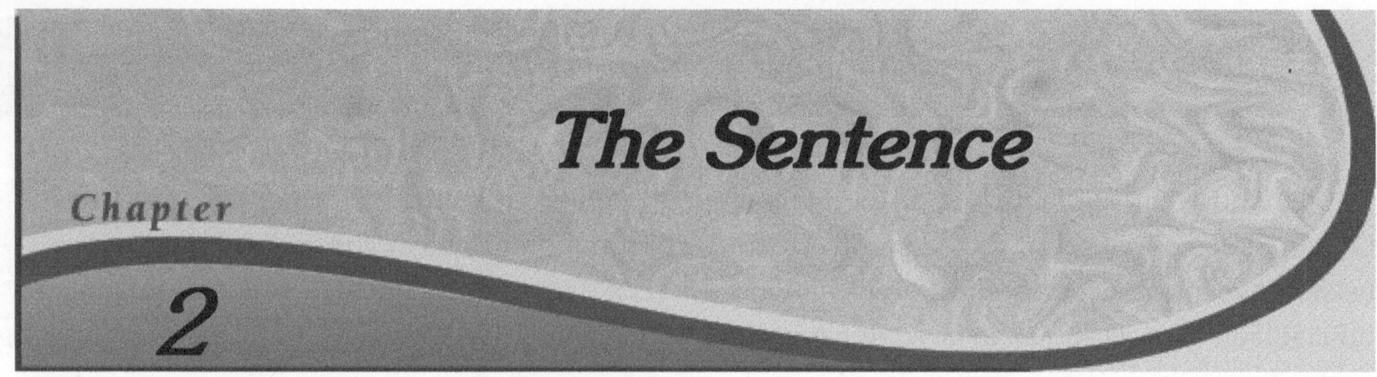


We all use words when we speak or write.

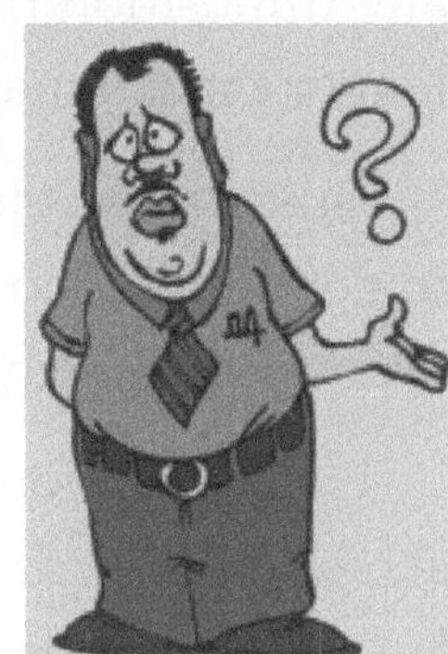

Now, here is an example of some words:

Car went Sameer church street madam bus

Tell me, do these words written in a line make sense? Why doesn't it make sense?

This is because they are just words written in a line and there is no connection between any of the words.

Now tell me few words which make sense or have meaning. In other words the words must be connected together.

This is a book on Nursing.

This makes complete sense. This is because the words tell us or give us some information. Every word is connected to give meaning.

A group of words which makes complete sense is called *a sentence.*

Now write five sentences.

1. ______________________________________________

2. ______________________________________________

3. ______________________________________________

4. ______________________________________________

5. ______________________________________________

# The Sentence

Just like different types of people, vehicles, we have different types of sentences. They are four in number.

### Type1

I am a senior nurse.

This makes a statement or it asserts what is in life. Such a sentence is called a **Declarative** or **Assertive sentence.**

### Type 2

Why did you disturb the doctor?

This asks a question. Such a sentence is called an **Interrogative sentence**.

### Type 3

Be silent.

Be kind to us.

Please shut the door.

These sentences show a command, request and an entreaty. Such sentences are called **Imperative sentences**.

### Type 4

Oh God! Show us some Mercy!

How cold it is outside!

It is shameful!

These sentences express strong feelings. Such sentences are called as **Exclamatory sentence** (They usually have an exclamatory mark).

## Exercise

**Identify the types of sentences given below:**

1. The sun sets in the west. ____________________
2. Where do you live? ____________________
3. Shut the door. ____________________
4. Help me please. ____________________
5. Oh no! She is bleeding! ____________________
6. Which state do you come from? ____________________
7. Pass the sutures. ____________________
8. Stand up straight. ____________________
9. May I come in? ____________________
10. Aah! I can't stand the pain. ____________________



## Parts of a Sentence

Just like we have different parts of a human body, we have parts of a sentence. When a sentence is made, it tells us—

i. about some person or thing, and

ii. says something about that person or thing.

*For example:*

1. Every nurse would have undergone training.
2. Sit down.

In the first sentence, we are speaking about a person and some information is given about this person.

# The Sentence

The portion which names the person or thing we are speaking about is called the ***Subject*** of the sentence.

The portion which tells something about the Subject is called the ***Predicate*** of the sentence.

Usually the subject of a sentence comes first. Sometimes, it is put after the predicate like

Down went the Titanic.

In the second sentence, we are dealing with Imperative sentence. Here the subject is left out.

Sit down. [*You* is the subject. It is understood.]

> ***Note:*** In orders, commands and requests generally the subject is left out.

No one says "You get out" or "You shut up your mouth."

## Exercise

**Identify the subject and the predicate in the following sentences:**

1. The singing of the birds delights us.
2. Solomon was rude at the church today.
3. They have a good memory.
4. Borrowed garments never fit well.
5. All roads lead to Rome.
6. Too many cooks spoil the broth.
7. A sick room should be well-aired.
8. The moon revolves round the sun.
9. The injection was given by me.
10. Head injuries are taken to Neuro-Science hospitals.

## Phrase and Clause

Now look at this group of words "on a wall".

It makes sense, but not complete sense. We need something added to this group of words to make complete sense.

Such a group of words which makes sense, but not complete sense, is called a ***Phrase***.

Now look at this group of words.

People *who pay their debts* are trusted.

This has a subject (who) and a predicate (pay their debts).

A group of words which forms part of a sentence, and contains a subject and a predicate, is called a ***Clause***.

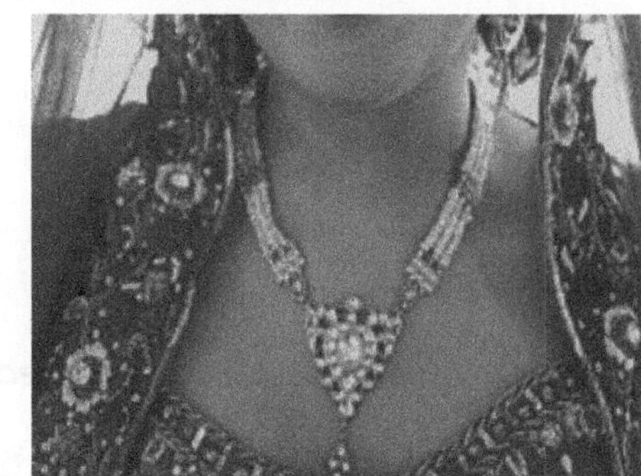



### *Examples for Phrases*

1. The sun sets *in the west*.
2. Show her *how to do it*.
3. She *let it go*.
5. Mother has a chain *of gold*.

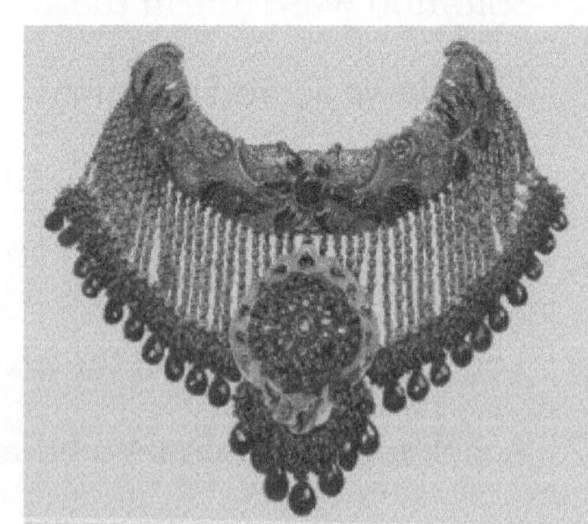

### *Examples for Clauses*

1. Mother has a chain *which is made of gold*.
2. Teacher thinks *that you have made a mistake*.

### Exercises

**I. Identify the phrases and clauses in the following sentences:**

1. You look *a bit* pale today.
2. I am not going home yet. My sister's *coming over* first.

3. I *look forward to* my first surgery session.
4. The lady *who lives next door* is a dentist.
5. Mohammed Waseem works for a company *that makes surgical equipments.*
6. The student nurses saw some people *whose car had broken down.*
7. *I expect* the professor of anatomy will extend the class.
8. It is tough *to settle down* in a boring job.
9. "I don't think my parents will be able to come. *It's a pity,* isn't it?"
10. An interior decorator is someone *who designs and decorates the insides of a building.*
11. I met somebody *whose mother writes nursing textbooks.*

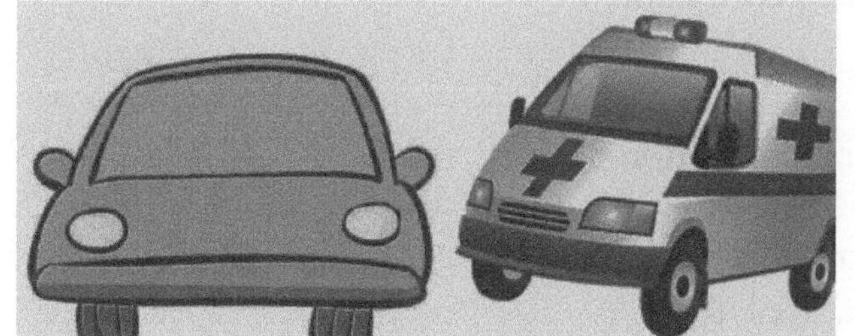

12. The old doctor went back to the town *where he was born.*
13. "Well, I must *get on* with my work."
14. The huge car was parked *in front of* the ambulance.

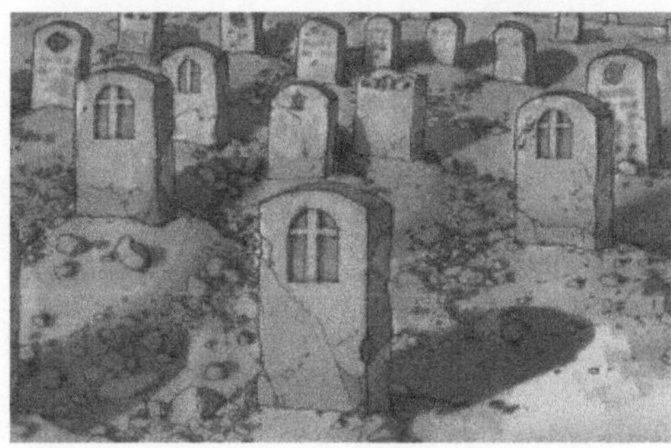

15. "I can't even sing the national anthem *in tune.*"
16. A cemetery is a place *where people are buried.*
17. Geetha has three brothers, *all of whom are doctors.*
18. Roger said, "They asked me a lot of questions, *most of which* I couldn't answer."
19. The house *where we stayed* wasn't very clean.
20. If I don't start studying now, I will *get into a muddle* during the exams.

**II. Try to form sentences of your own for the following phrases:**

i. If I were

ii. the last straw

iii. after a time

iv. ask (somebody *) to tea

v. happen to be

vi. a couple of

vii. in addition

viii. look for

ix. ring (somebody *) up

x. at all

* Replace this with a name or a pronoun.

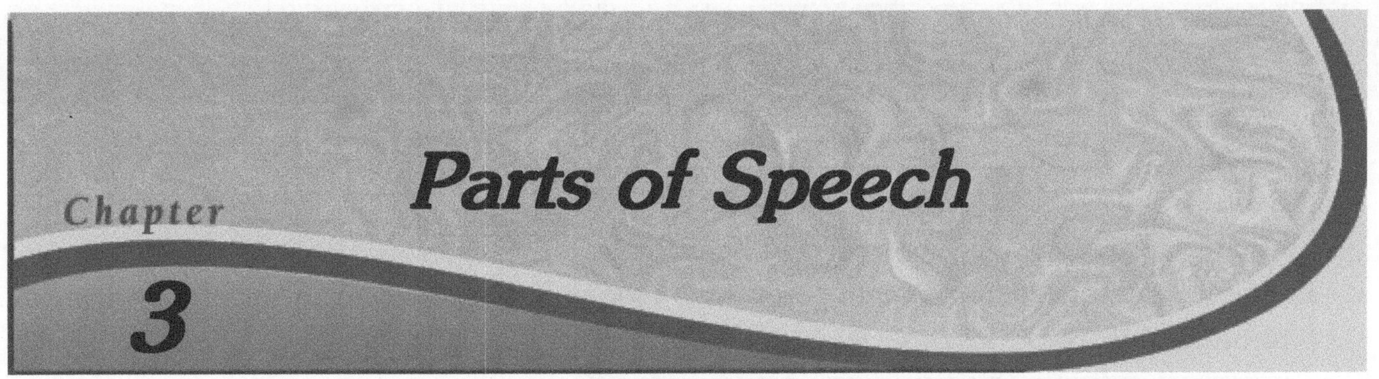

# Chapter 3 Parts of Speech

When we talk or when we write, we use words. Some of them describe a person, place, thing or event. Some show action, some more add emphasis to the description. There will be words which have the names of people or places. All these words that we use, fall into different categories. In other words, words are divided into different kinds called Parts of Speech. Just as different parts of a body serve a specific purpose, Parts of Speech serves a specific purpose in conversation or while reading.

The words based on the work they do in a sentence are divided into eight specific parts. They are:

1. Noun
2. Adjective
3. Pronoun
4. Verb
5. Adverb
6. Preposition
7. Conjunction
8. Interjection

1. ***A Noun:*** This is a word used as the name of a person, place, or thing.

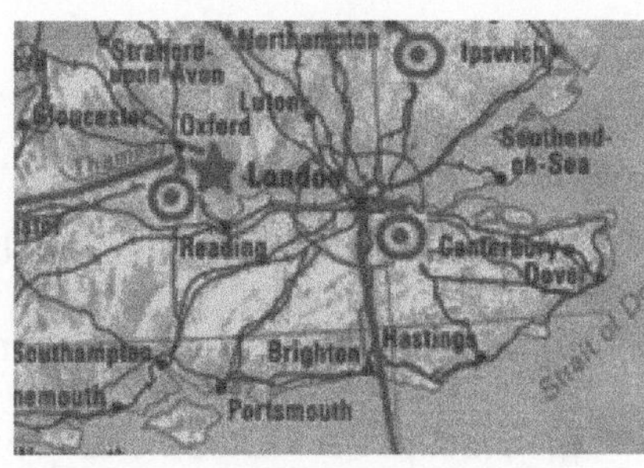


*Example:*

*i. Chandra Gupta Maurya* was a great king.

*ii London* is on the banks of *Thames.*

*iii.* The *Jasmine* smells *sweet.*

*iv.* The *moon* shines *silvery.*

*v.* Their *courage* won them *honour.*

> **Note:** The word thing includes all objects that we can see, hear, taste, touch or smell and something that we can think of; but cannot perceieve by the senses–idea, dream, imagination.

2. ***An Adjective***: This is a word used to add something to the meaning of a noun.

   *Example:*

   i. He is a *handsome man*.

   ii. There are *fifty* nursing students in *this* class.

3. ***A Pronoun***: This is a word used instead of a noun.

   *Example:*

   i. Mary is absent, because *she* is ill.

   ii. The papers are where you left *them*.



4. ***A Verb***: This is a word used to *say* something about some person, place or thing. Since it shows work being done, it is also called as Action word.

   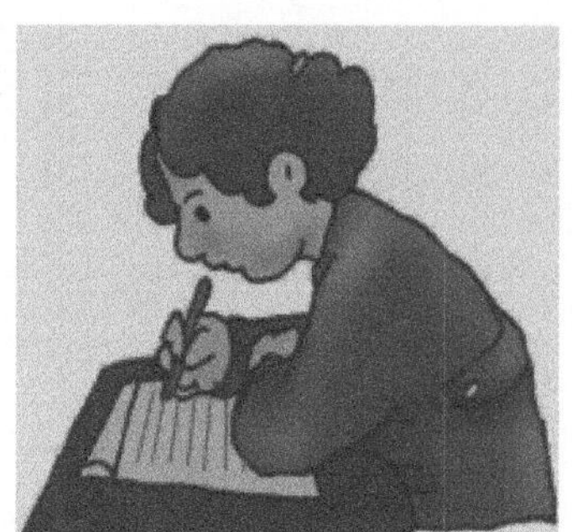

   *Example:*

   i. The student *wrote* a letter to the Principal.

   ii. Bengaluru *is* a big city.

   Penicillin injections *save* many lives.

5. ***An Adverb***: This is a word used to *add something* to the meaning of a verb, an adjective or another adverb.

   *Example:*

   i. The nurse gave the injection *quickly*.

   ii. That bouquet is *very beautiful*.

   iii. Sam pronounced the word *quite* correctly.

6. ***A Preposition:*** This is a word used with a noun or a pronoun to show how the person or thing denoted by the noun or pronoun stands in relation to something else.

   *Example:*

   i. The *students* are sitting *inside* the class.
   (Noun)

   ii. *Everyone* is fond *of* music.
   (Pronoun)

   *iii. Mini* is sitting *under* a tree.
   (Noun)

   Here students, Mini are nouns; everyone is a pronoun.

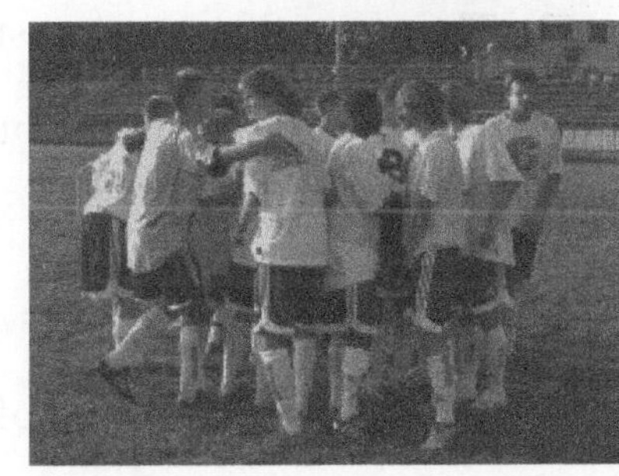

7. ***A Conjunction:*** This is a word used to *join* words or sentences.

   *Example:*

   i. Adeena *and* Rekha are friends.

   ii. One *and* one makes two.

   iii. They ran fast, *but* missed the bus.

8. ***An Interjection:*** This is a word which expresses some sudden feeling.

   *Example:*

   i. Cheers! We did it.

   ii. Alas! The doctor could not save her.

> ***Note:*** It is necessary for us to understand that the words are divided into different clauses according to the work they do in a sentence. But, we cannot say to which part of speech a word belongs unless we see it used in a sentence.

*Example:* `After' is a word, when we use it in the following sentences we observe how the Parts of Speech change.

i. They arrived soon *after*. ( Adverb)

ii. They arrived *after* us. (Preposition)

iii. They arrived *after* we had left. (Conjunction)

## Exercise

**Name the part of speech of each italicized word in the following sentences.**

1. *Bengaluru* is a metropolitan city.
2. There are *fifty* nursing students in this class.
3. All the nurses sat in a bus. *They* were taken to a hospital from *their* College.
4. The doctors *treated* the patients with diarrhea.
5. They climbed the stairs *quickly*.
6. The box is *under* the table.
7. Harry bought rice *but* forgot to get sugar.
8. *Hurray*! We won.
9. The doctor's *courage* won him *honour*.
10. A pair of scissors is used to cut the paper *quickly*.
11. *He* refused to take the tablet.
12. He *sang* well.
13. The labour pains came *very* fast with less time duration.
14. We walk *on* the footpath.
15. Jyotsna *and* Abida study together.
16. *Yahoo*! We are going to see snowfall in Kashmir.
17. A *bouquet* was given to the best nurse.
18. A trolley is *wheeled* fast in an emergency.
19. It is a *well* designed hospital.
20. Reshma, Sushila and Jacob went *to shop* for aprons.

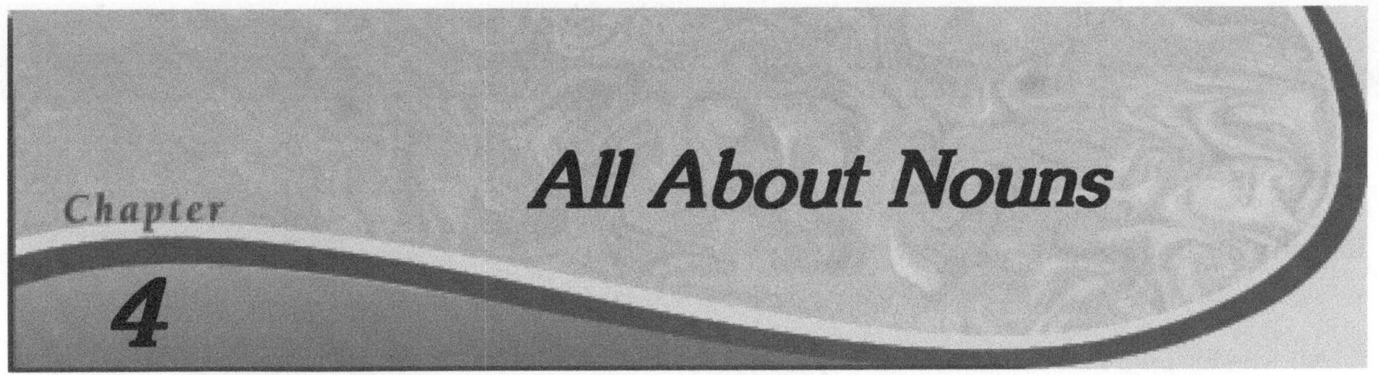


## Definition

A Noun is a word which is used as the name of a person, place or thing. It is also used in titles or ranks that people hold.

It is to be noted that *thing* is used to mean anything that we can *think of.*

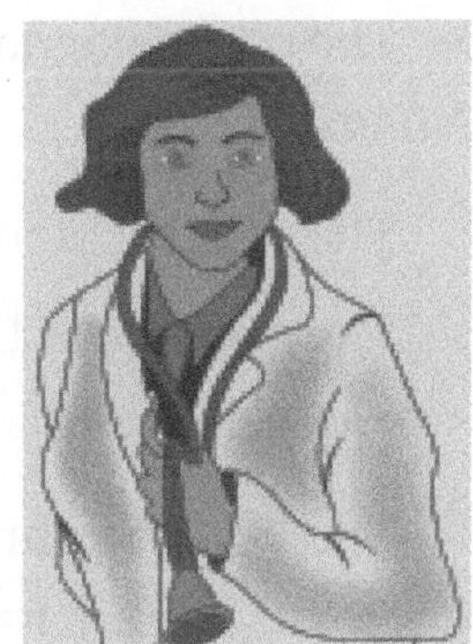

Let us take the following examples:

1. *Shobha* is a famous *doctor*.
2. *Robert* is a *boy*.
3. *India* is a *country*.
4. *Asia* is a *continent*.

   Here Shobha, Robert , India, Asia are particular names of people and places.
   Doctor, boy, *country*, continent are general names given to persons or places of the same kind.

Now consider these examples:

1. The *crowd* shouted for *justice*.
2. The *team* played *bravely* in the rain.
3. An *army* of ants is *interesting* to watch.
4. A *flock* flew towards the *bright* sunlight.

Here crowd, team, army, flock are a collection of people and birds (flock). While justice, bravely, interesting, bright are feelings that cannot be touched.

All these examples denote nouns.

## Exercise

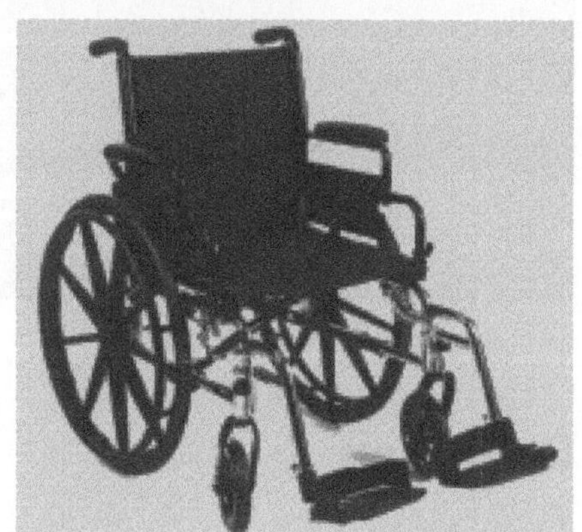

**Identify the nouns here.**

1. Denmark is in Europe.
2. Middle East is a favourite destination for nurses.
3. Roshan is a foolish man.
4. The wheel-chair is needed in a hospital.
5. Earlier, syringes were sterilized before every use.

All the above examples also show different kinds of nouns.

The particular names in the previous examples like Shobha, Robert, India, and Asia are called ***Proper Nouns***.

The general identity like doctor, boy, *country*, and continent are called ***Common Nouns***.

The collections like crowd, team, army, flock are called ***Collective Nouns***.

The feelings like justice, bravely, interesting are called ***Abstract Nouns***.

The noun Shobha refers to a particular person but the noun doctor may be applied to any other doctor as well as to Shobha. Therefore Shobha is a proper noun and doctor is a common noun. *Same way, the noun India refers to a particular place but the noun country may be applied to any city including India.*

### *Definitions*

***Proper Noun:*** Is the name of a particular person or place.

***Common Noun:*** Is the name given in common to every person or thing of the same kind .

***Collective Noun:*** Is the name of a number of persons or things taken together and spoken as one whole.

***Abstract Noun:*** Is the name of a quality, action or state considered apart from the object to which it belongs.

*Example:*

1. Quality–Goodness, kindness
2. Action–Laughter, theft
3. State–Childhood, youth

**The names of subjects like Arts and Science (grammar, music, Physics) are also Abstract nouns.**

***Material Noun:*** Is the name of a substance or material.

*Example:* Copper, iron, tin

***Note # 1:*** Proper nouns are always written with a capital letter at the beginning.

***Note # 2:*** Abstract nouns can be formed from adjectives (kindness from kind), verbs (obedience from obey) and common nouns (childhood from child).

**Remember**

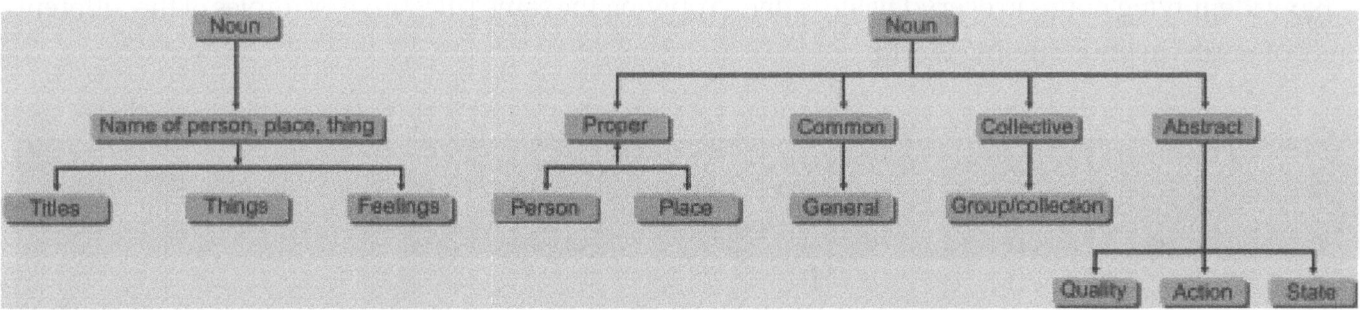




## Exercise

**Identify the Nouns by underlining them and classify them as common, proper, collective or abstract:**

1. Cleanliness is next to godliness.
2. Dr Reeta is a well-known gynecologist.
3. The Brahmaputra overflows its banks every year.
4. Dr Rowena is a senior surgeon.
5. Always speak the truth.
6. Mathematics is not taught in Medical Colleges.
7. Dr Subrahmanya is a professor Emeritus.
8. Nandita and Aradhya are the assisting nurses in the operation theatre today.

9. A committee of eight was appointed yesterday.
10. The class is studying grammar.
11. This room is fifty feet in length.
12. We all think of the happy days of childhood.
13. I recognized your voice at once.
14. Never tell a lie.
15. Wisdom is better than strength.

Now identifying nouns in everyday life is fine. Applying the same rules, give examples of the different kinds of nouns in your nursing world:



| Proper Nouns | | Common Nouns | Abstract Nouns | Collective Nouns |
|---|---|---|---|---|
| Person | Place | | | |
| 1. | | | | |
| 2. | | | | |
| 3. | | | | |
| 4. | | | | |
| 5. | | | | |
| 6. | | | | |
| 7. | | | | |
| 8. | | | | |
| 9. | | | | |
| 10. | | | | |

# All About Nouns

Earlier we studied that abstract nouns can be formed from adjectives, verbs and common nouns. Let us see how to do it.

First let us take forming abstract nouns from adjectives. (Remember adjectives are describing words).

| Adjectives | | Abstract Nouns | |
|---|---|---|---|
| long | describes measurement | length | But these can only be experienced. None of these can be touched. |
| strong | describes the capacity of a person or object. | strength | |
| wide | describes space available | width | |
| broad | describes measurement | breadth | |
| high | describes vertical measurement | height | |

Similarly, change these words now:

| Adjectives | Abstract Nouns |
|---|---|
| young | ______________ |
| true | ______________ |
| wise | ______________ |
| free | ______________ |
| poor | ______________ |
| humble | ______________ |
| decent | ______________ |
| cruel | ______________ |
| bitter | ______________ |
| short | ______________ |

Next let us take forming abstract nouns from verbs. (Remember verbs are action words.)

| Verbs | Abstract Nouns |
| --- | --- |
| Laugh–Action of smiling and sound being produced. | Laughter–Can be heard |
| Believe | Belief |
| Defend | Defence |

Similarly change these words now:

| Verbs | Abstract Nouns |
| --- | --- |
| obey | ______________ |
| live | ______________ |
| expect | ______________ |
| excel | ______________ |
| known | ______________ |
| serve | ______________ |
| hate | ______________ |
| seize | ______________ |
| flatter | ______________ |
| discover | ______________ |

Next let us take forming abstract nouns from common nouns.

| Common Nouns | Abstract Nouns |
| --- | --- |
| king | kinghood/kingship- process of being king. |
| man | manhood |
| thief | thievery |
| mother | motherhood |
| glutton | gluttony |

Similarly, change these words now:

| Common Nouns | Abstract Nouns |
|---|---|
| infant | ______________ |
| priest | ______________ |
| author | ______________ |
| friend | ______________ |
| agent | ______________ |
| woman | ______________ |
| author | ______________ |
| pirate | ______________ |
| beggar | ______________ |
| bond | ______________ |

All this is fine. How does one connect all this to the medical life the nursing students face? Here is a case history. Identify the nouns given in the case study. Underline the nouns and write the type of noun identified.

## Case History

Radha was at the nursing station at August Nursing Home. She was waiting to go off duty. Just at that moment a couple walked into the hospital. They were directed to meet nurse Radha. She quickly understood that the man required medical assistance. She quickly asked questions. She found that a continued stomach pain along with vomiting five times had brought the couple to the hospital. She continued to ask questions and started recording the man's answers. Occasionally, the wife would add points. She took his temperature which was normal. The sphygmomanometer gave his blood pressure to be slightly high. His pulse rate was recorded. She then checked his weight and height. He weighed 70 kgs, when he stood on the weighing machine. The complaint of ringing in the ears was made by him. When asked, the man said his name to be Sandesh Bhat. Mrs Sharada Bhat told the nurse that he had a past history of ear infection, but the ENT surgeon Dr Ali Khan had helped in curing it. To meet Dr Ali they had travelled to Hyderabad by plane a few years earlier. Mrs Bhat softly added that the problem had begun after Mr Bhat ate some Thai food which he was not used to. The various instruments in the nursing station made Mr Bhat wish to just go away from all these white-coated people. He looked gloomy. Nurse Radha recorded all this and now she felt she could send them to Dr Solomon with the details she had recorded. By this time nurse Edwina came to relieve nurse Radha. She waited for Radha to come out of the consultation room. Before Radha left for home, she briefed nurse Edwina about the work and the patient who had come in.

1. ______________________________

______________________________

2. ______________________________

______________________________



3. ______________________________

______________________________

4. ______________________________

______________________________

5. ______________________________

______________________________

6. ______________________________

## Noun: Gender

From kinds of Noun, we come to an important topic in Nouns. It is called Noun: Gender. We all know living beings are either of male or female sex.

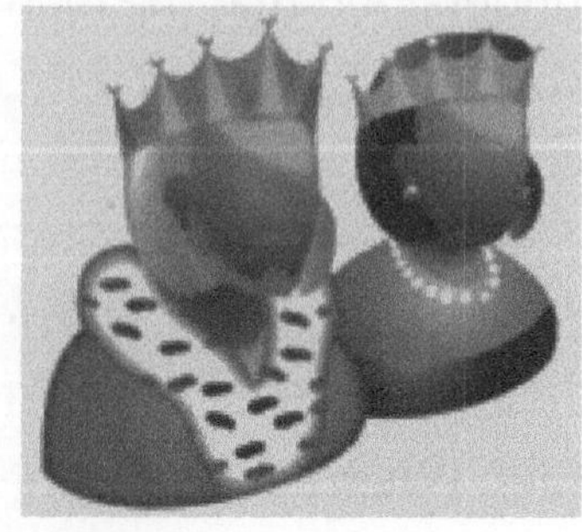

| *For example:* | King | Tiger | Pea-cock |
|---|---|---|---|
| | Queen | Tigress | Pea-hen |

The words in the first line shows a male animal or bird.

*Definition:* A noun which shows a *male living being* is said to be the **Masculine gender**.

The words in the second line show a female animal or bird.

*Definition:* A noun which shows a *female living being* is said to be the **Feminine gender**.

> ***Note:*** Gender is got from the Latin word *genus* which means kind or sort

*Definition:* A noun which shows either a male or a female is said to be **Common gender**.

*Example:* Parent, teacher, friend, ruler, neighbour, person, cousin, baby

*Definition:* A noun which shows a thing that is *neither male nor female* is said to be **Neuter gender**. That is it denotes a thing without life.

*Example:* Book, pen, tree, table, paper, stethoscope, forceps.

*Note #1.* Collective nouns though they may denote living beings, are considered as Neuter- gender.

*Example:* Bouquet, cluster (a group of stars)

*Note #2.* Young children and lower animals are also classified under neuter gender.

Some Grammar books classify Genders based on how they are formed. Some books don't have any classification. But, we will follow a classification for easy learning and recalling what we learn.

Genders are classified usually in the following manner:

I. By using entirely different word:

| **Masculine** | **Feminine** |
|---|---|
| Boy | Girl |
| King | Queen |
| Cock | Hen |
| Dog | Bitch |
| Lord | Lady |
| Man | Woman |

II. By adding -ess, -ine, -trix, a to the word:

| **Masculine** | **Feminine** |
|---|---|
| Author | Authoress |

| | |
|---|---|
| Priest | Priestess |
| Hero | Heroine |
| Administrator | Administratrix |
| Czar * | Czarina* |

(* Russian King and Queen)

III. By placing a word before the word or after:

| **Masculine** | **Feminine** |
|---|---|
| He-goat | She-goat |
| Man-servant | Maid-servant |

## Exercises

**I. Identify the gender of the following words:**

1. Brother
2. Sister
3. Sir
4. Stag
5. Wizard
6. Vixen
7. Key
8. Principal
9. Commander
10. Surgeon
11. Helper
12. Trolley
13. Gas-mask
14. Patient

15. Doctor
16. Sultana
17. Land-lord
18. Compounder
19. Lab-assistant
20. Singer

**II. Fill in the blanks with the correct form of the gender:**

| | Masculine | Feminine |
|---|---|---|
| 1. | Bull (or ox) | _______ |
| 2. | _______ | Filly |
| 3. | Drake | _______ |
| 4. | _______ | Bee |
| 5. | Earl | _______ |
| 6. | Father | _______ |
| 7. | _______ | Goose |
| 8. | Host | _______ |
| 9. | Lion | _______ |
| 10. | _______ | Manageress |
| 11. | _______ | Mayoress |
| 12. | Poet | _______ |
| 13. | Founder | _______ |
| 14. | Shepherd | _______ |
| 15. | Actor | _______ |
| 16. | _______ | Negress |

17. _______ Duchess

18. _______ Princess

19. Grand-father _______

20. Milk-man _______

21. Inventor _______

The next topic in Nouns is the noun number.

## The Noun Number

This helps us in denoting the quantity of a word.

Let us take these pair of words:

| Boy | Girl | Ox | Woman | Man |
|---|---|---|---|---|
| Boys | Girls | Oxen | Women | Men |

The first line denotes one thing of each noun.

The second line denotes more than one thing of each noun.

A noun which shows one person or thing is called **Singular Number**.

A noun which shows more than one person or thing is called **Plural Number.**

When we take the word pairs above, we see that the plurals are formed in different ways. 's' is not always added to show more than one noun or person, like–

| Man | Ox | Man | Ox |
|---|---|---|---|
| Mans × | Oxs × | Men ✓ | Oxen✓ |

This leads us to the question how are plurals formed?

There are certain rules to be followed while forming plurals. There are six major rules. If we follow these, we cannot go wrong in forming plurals of different words.

*Rule 1.* A plural is generally formed by adding -s to the singular.

| *Like* | Boy | Girl | Table | Pen | Dog |
|---|---|---|---|---|---|
| | Boys | Girls | Tables | Pens | Dogs |

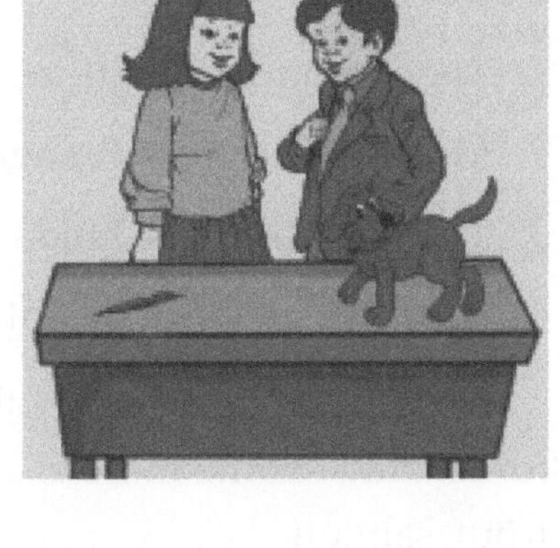

*Rule 2.* If the noun ends in -s, -sh, -ch or -x, plurals are formed by adding -es to the singular.

| *Like* | Class | Brush | Match | Box |
|---|---|---|---|---|
| | Classes | Brushes | Matches | Boxes |

*Rule 3.* Most nouns ending in -o also have plurals formed by adding -es to the singular.

| *Like* | Buffalo | Potato | Mango |
|---|---|---|---|
| | Buffaloes | Potatoes | Mangoes |

*Rule 4.* A few nouns ending in -o, generally those which are in less usage form plurals by just adding -s.

| *Like* | Dynamo | Piano | Photo |
|---|---|---|---|
| | Dynamos | Pianos | Photos |

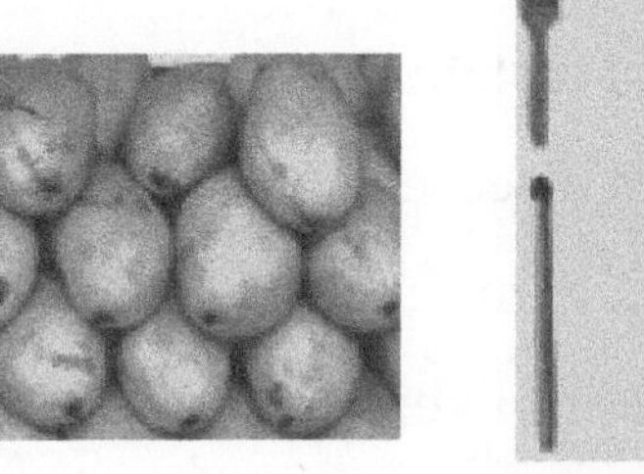

*Rule 5.* Nouns which end in -y and are preceded by a consonant, form plurals by changing -y into i, then -es is added.

| *Like* | Baby | Army | Story |
|---|---|---|---|
| | Babies | Armies | Stories |

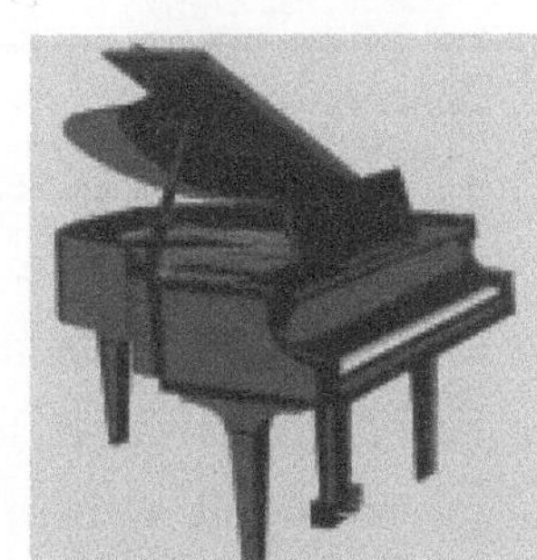

*Rule 6.* Nouns ending in -f or -fe form plurals by changing -f or -fe into 'v' and then -es is added.

| *Like* | Thief | Life | Loaf | Wife |
|---|---|---|---|---|
| | Thieves | Lives | Loaves | Wives |

NOTE: There are some exceptions to this rule. Like–

| Chief | Roof | Dwarf |
|---|---|---|
| Chiefs | Roofs | Dwarfs |

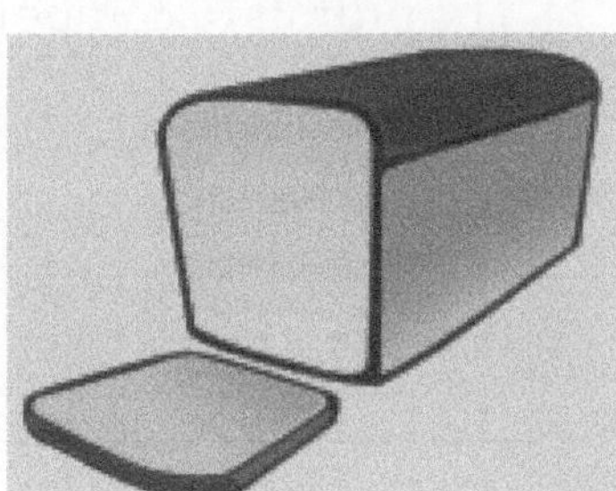

A few plurals are formed by changing the inside vowel of the singular :

| Man | Mouse | Foot |
|---|---|---|
| Men | Mice | Feet |

Chapter 4

Observe these sentences.

1. The visitors bought three *dozen* mangoes.
2. Most people reach the age of three *score* and ten these days.
3. The operation cost Linda four *thousand* dollars.
4. Atilla weighs above eight *stone.*

Here these nouns have both the singular and plural forms alike. Some more examples are–swine, deer, trout, salmon.

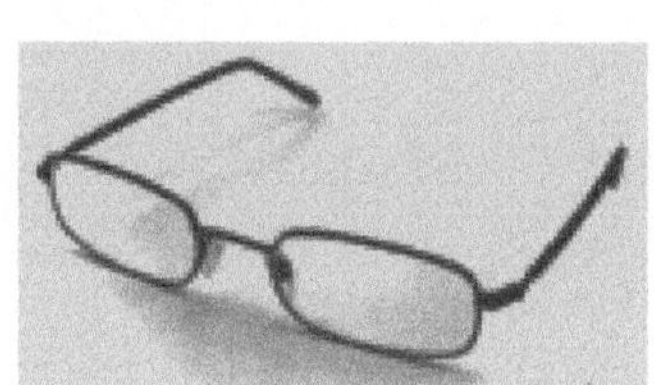

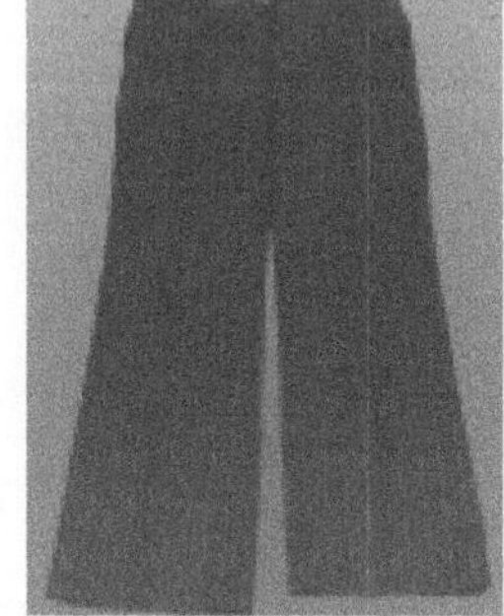

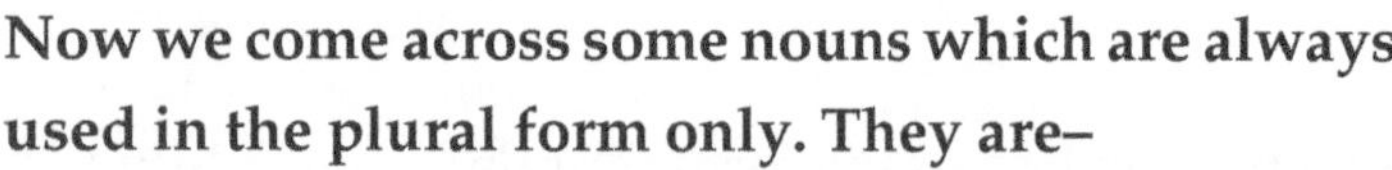

**Now we come across some nouns which are always used in the plural form only. They are–**

i. Names of instruments: Forceps, scissors, spectacles.
ii. Names of certain dresses: Trousers, drawers, knickers.
iii. Names of diseases: Measles, mumps.
iv. Names of games: Billiards.
v. Other nouns like: Thanks, tidings, nuptials

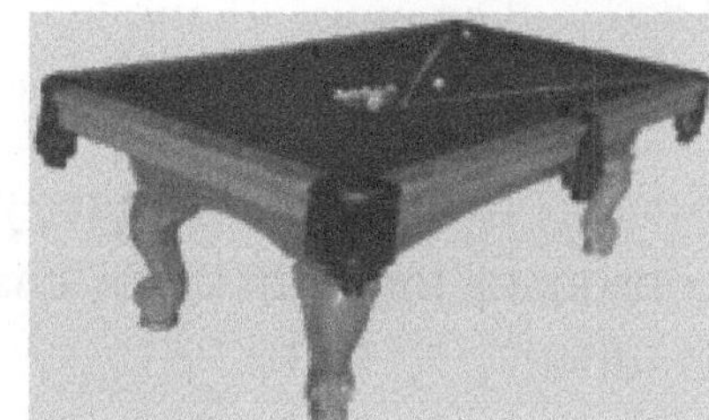



*Note:*

1. Names of diseases are classified under abstract nouns. This is because living beings can experience diseases but cannot touch a disease all by itself like the other nouns. Thus there are no singular or plural to diseases. Ex. (iii) gives the spelling in plural. There are no singular forms for these.
2. Names of subjects like Mathematics, Physics, Politics, News do not have singular or plural form. The spelling is in plural form. But the names of subjects are used in singular form in speech and in writing.

The plurals of compound nouns are formed by adding -s to the principal word, like–

| | |
|---|---|
| Son-in-law | Sons-in-law |
| Step-son | Step-sons |
| Commander-in-chief | Commanders-in-Chief |
| Ward-boy | Ward-boys |

## What are Compound Nouns?

These are nouns formed when two different words are combined to give a word with a different meaning altogether.

*Example:* Pea and cock combine to give pea-cock.

Pea is a vegetable. Cock is a bird. Together they give a different word. Pea-cock that is a different bird.

Grand+father=grandfather (oldman or father's father or mother's father)

## Exercises

**I. Give the plural forms of the following nouns. If it does not exist, mark ×:**

| | | | |
|---|---|---|---|
| desk | ____________ | pony | ____________ |
| trout | ____________ | lady | ____________ |
| cow | ____________ | city | ____________ |
| brush | ____________ | cod | ____________ |
| kiss | ____________ | safe | ____________ |
| tax | ____________ | brief | ____________ |
| volcano | ____________ | hoof | ____________ |
| hero | ____________ | strife | ____________ |
| echo | ____________ | goose | ____________ |
| solo | ____________ | woman | ____________ |
| memento | ____________ | tooth | ____________ |
| stereo | ____________ | breeches | ____________ |
| pair | ____________ | pincers | ____________ |
| hundred | ____________ | annals | ____________ |
| tongs | ____________ | fish | ____________ |
| draughts | ____________ | penny | ____________ |
| coat-of-mail | ____________ | maid-servant | ____________ |

**II. Identify the different types of nouns in this passage:**

During the seventeenth century there were great developments in the spheres of human knowledge other than medicine and chemistry. This did have its impact on future developments in the field of chemotherapy. It was the age of physics and mathematics, the age of giants like Galileo, Newton, Kepler, Locke, Bacon and Spinoza: Men who contributed to the development of experimental science. No less important was the construction of the tiny microscope by the Dutch cloth merchant, Antonie von Leeuwenhoek, and his observation of the tiny animals; suddenly, the until-then-unknown bacteria were discovered.

______________________________________________

______________________________________________

______________________________________________

______________________________________________

______________________________________________



**III. Fill in the blanks with the appropriate forms of singular and plural of the nouns given in the brackets:**

In the year 1796, Edward Jenner took some __________ (pus/puses) from Cowpox __________ (eruption/eruptions) in the __________ (hand) of a __________ (milk-maid/milk-maids) called Sarah Nelmes and inserted it by two superficial __________ (incision/incisions) into the __________ (arm/arms) of James Philipps, an eight-year old ________ (boy/boys). This was the first __________ (vaccination/vaccinations) in history. Two ________ (month/months) later, virulent small pox matter was injected by Jenner into the boy's ________ (arm/arms).

The boy did not contract smallpox and remained completely unaffected by the __________ (injection/injections). The boy had acquired __________ (immunity/immunities) to __________ (smallpox/smallpoxes).

## Countable and Uncountable Nouns

Nouns can be countable or uncountable. They are denoted by the short form C and U. That is some nouns can be easily quantified. In other words, some nouns that are present, their number is easy to know. There are some nouns whose number present cannot be found out at all.

# All About Nouns

See these sentences.

- An apple a day keeps the doctor away.
- The hospital canteen buys 40 kgs of rice every month.
- I like apples.
- South Indians like rice.

Here apple, doctor, hospital are countable nouns whereas rice cannot be counted. None can count the grains of rice.

You can see that countable nouns can have singular or plural form. Uncountable nouns have only one form.

Compare the two sets of sentences:

| Countable | Uncountable |
|---|---|
| • Goa has good *beaches*. | • There's *sand* in all our shoes. |
| • Pradeep is singing a *song*. | • Pradeep loves to *listen* to music. |
| • What is your *Hb count*? | • *Blood* poured out of the wound. |
| • Throw the dead *batteries*. | • There is no *electricity* in Bengaluru today. |

In the above sentences, beaches, song hemoglobin count and batteries can all be counted and we do get to know the number or the reading of the said noun.

In the above sentences sand, listen, blood, and electricity are too intangible to count. It is impossible to attempt to count any of these. Thus uncountable nouns represent huge quantities or forces in nature.

A few more examples are–

***Countable Nouns:*** Wheelchair, thermometer, stethoscope, coat

***Uncountable Nouns:*** Solution, saliva, anger, humility

## Exercises

**I. Write C for countable noun or U for uncountable noun in the space provided:**

1. Watch ____________________
2. Pericardium ____________________

3. Colostrum ____________________
4. Decrudescence ____________________
5. Elbow ____________________
6. Decomposition ____________________
7. Uniform ____________________
8. Feeling ____________________
9. Lancet ____________________
10. Microtome ____________________



**II. Fill in the blanks with the appropriate nouns (Countable or Uncountable) given in the brackets:**

1. ____________ belong to the hospital. (These chairs, Chair)
2. We had a lot of ________________. (baggage, luggage)
3. The matron gave a good ____________. (suggestions, suggestion)
4. The senior surgeon Mr Rao gave good ____________. (advice, advise)
5. Nobody was hurt in the accident but the ____________ (damage, damages) to the car ___________ (was, were) quite bad.

# Chapter 5

# All About Adjectives

We come across sentences like these in our daily lives.

1. Abheesh is a *clever* nurse.
2. Adeena doesn't like *that* doctor.
3. Varghese gave the patient *two* bananas.
4. Nurse Dona told nurse Sebastian "*Not much* time left for us to dash into the lecture hall."

In the first sentence *clever* shows *what* kind of boy Abheesh is.

In the second sentence *that* points out *which* doctor is meant.

In the third sentence *two* shows *how many* bananas Varghese gave the patient.

In the fourth sentence *not much* shows *how much* time there is for preparation.

These words 'clever', 'that', 'two', 'not much' describe or point out the noun (person, animal, place or thing). In other words, they tell us the number or quality of the noun. Such words are called **Adjectives**.

*Definition:* Adjective is a word used with a noun to add something for its meaning.

OR

Adjective is a word used to describe a noun.

## Kinds of Adjectives

There are seven different kinds of Adjectives.
They are:

1. Adjectives of Quality (or Descriptive Adjectives)
2. Adjectives of Quantity

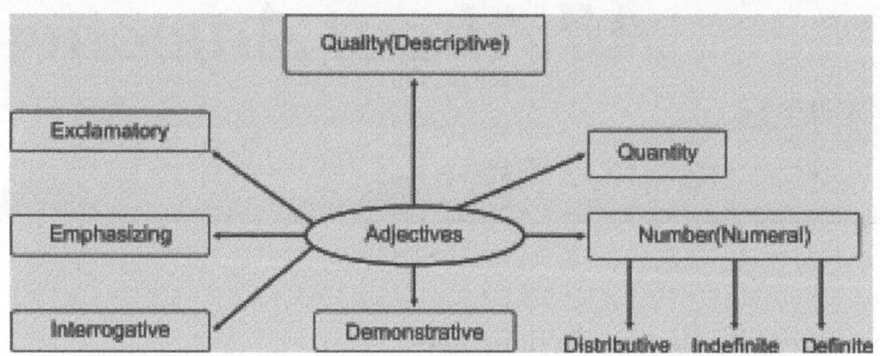


3. Adjectives of Number (or Numeral Adjectives)
4. Demonstrative Adjectives
5. Interrogative Adjectives
6. Emphasizing Adjectives
7. Exclamatory Adjectives



## *Definitions*

1. **Adjectives of Quality (or Descriptive Adjectives):** These are words which show the kind or quality of a person or thing. It answers the question *of what kind?*

   *Example:*

   i. Om Hospital is a *large* hospital.

   ii. Azimudeen is an *honest* nurse.

   iii. *French** wines are world *famous*.

   iv. This is a Grammar of the *English** Language.

   [*Adjectives formed from Proper Nouns are called Proper Adjectives. They are put with Adjectives of Quality.]

2. **Adjectives of Quantity:** These are words which show *how much* a thing is present or meant. It answers the question *How much*?

   *Example:*

   i. Varghese ate *some* rice in the hospital canteen.

ii. Nurse Rekha showed *much* patience.

iii. Dr Sowmya used *little* intelligence in calming the patient.

iv. The obese man had *enough* exercise today.

v. Matron Mary lost *all* her money.

vi. Take *great care* of your health.

3. **Adjectives of Number:** These are words which show how many persons or things are present or meant or *in what* order (or rank) a person or thing stands. It answers the question *how many*?

   *Example:*

   i. There are *five* toes on our foot.

   ii. *Few* old people can bear cold water bath.

   iii. There are *no* pictures in that book.

   iv. *All* humans must die.

   v. Sunday is the *first* day of the week.

   *Adjectives of Number are of three kinds. They are:*

   i. Definite Numeral Adjectives

   ii. Indefinite Numeral Adjectives

   iii. Distributive Numeral Adjectives

i. ***Definite Numeral Adjectives:*** These are words which denote an exact number.

   *Example:*

   One, two, three, ……. This kind of writing numbers is called Cardinal.

   First, second, …… This kind of writing the order of numbers is called Ordinals.

ii. ***Indefinite Numeral Adjectives:*** These are words which do not denote an exact number.

   *Example:* All, no, many, few, some, any, certain, several, etc.

iii. ***Distributive Numeral Adjectives:*** These are words which refer to each one of a number.

   *Example:*

   i. *Each* nurse must learn to give injection.

ii. *Either* pencil will do.

iii. *Neither* diagnosis is true.

iv. *Every* child is naughty.

At this point a few of you students may remember the examples of Adjectives of Quantity and say that examples of Adjectives of Numbers are the same. This does happen if you see just the words themselves. The usage differs. Look at these sentences:

| Adjectives of Quantity | Adjectives of Number |
|---|---|
| I ate *some* rice. | *Some* boys are clever. |
| You have *no* sense. | There are *no* pictures in that book. |
| Afzah has *enough* salt. | The college kitchen does not have *enough* spoons. |

Read the definitions and see the difference in the usage of the two kinds of adjectives. Your confusion will be eliminated.



4. **Demonstrative Adjectives:** These are words which point out/show in particular which person or thing is meant. It answers the question *which*?

*Example:*

i. *This* patient is stronger than the patient in bed 21.

ii. *That* nurse is industrious.

iii. *These* grapes are sour.

iv. Don't be in *such* a hurry.

> **Note:** *'This' and 'that' are used with Singular Nouns*
> *These* and *those* are used with Plural Nouns.

5. **Interrogative Adjectives:** These are words used with nouns to ask questions like *what, which* and *whose.*

*Example:*

i. *What* manner of a doctor is he?

ii. *Which* laboratory should we go into?

iii. *Whose* psychology books are these?

6. **Emphasizing Adjectives:** The two words *own* and *very* are used to give extra confirmation about an incident or thing. They are then called **Emphasizing Adjectives**.

*Example:*

i. I saw the accident happen with my *own* eyes.

ii. Mind your *own business*.

iii. That is the *very* thing we want.

7. **Exclamatory Adjectives:** The word *'what'* is sometimes used to show emotion- exclaiming over a happening/situation. At such times it is called as **Exclamatory Adjective**.

*Example:*

i. *What* intelligence! Here this is usually used sarcastically:

*What* genius! This gives a positive thought usually.

ii. *What* an idea!

iii. *What* a blessing! We have Dr Sudhir in surgery today.



## Exercise

**Identify the different kinds of adjectives italicized in the sentences given below:**

1. This is a Grammar of the *English* language.
2. He has *no* sense.
3. The patient in ward 3 did not eat *any* rice.

4. There has not been *sufficient* rain this year.
5. The head nurse taught the junior nurses *many* things.
6. Here are *some ripe* bananas.
7. *Most* boys like to get dirty.
8. A bird in the hand is worth *two* in the bush.
9. "There are *several* mistakes in your nursing notes" said the senior.
10. *Too many* cooks spoil the broth.
11. On *either* side the stones block the way.
12. The *first* patient to come in today is a hypochondriac.
13. The *hundredth* episode of the serial was boring.
14. *Those* rascals must be punished.
15. She is her *own* mistress.
16. *What* happiness!
17. *Which* way shall we go?
18. He is a man of *few* words.
19. Haseena secured the *second* rank in nursing exams.
20. The child fell down from a *great* height.



## Formation of Adjectives

In Chapter 4–All about Nouns, we studied how abstract nouns are formed from adjectives, verbs and common nouns. The same way, adjectives are formed from nouns, some from verbs and some are formed from other adjectives. Yes. You read right. Adjectives are formed from other adjectives.

i. Adjectives formed from Nouns:

| *Nouns* | *Adjectives* |
|---|---|
| Boy | Boyish |
| Fool | Foolish |
| Play | Playful |
| Trouble | Troublesome |
| Man | Manly |
| Shame | Shameless |
| Silk | Silken |
| Dirt | Dirty |
| Laugh | Laughable |
| Courage | Courageous |

ii. Adjectives formed from Verbs:

| *Verbs* | *Adjectives* |
|---|---|
| Tire | Tireless |
| Move | Movable |
| Talk | Talkative |

iii. Adjectives formed from other Adjectives:

| *Adjectives* | *Adjectives* |
|---|---|
| Tragic | Tragical |
| Whole | Wholesome |
| Three | Threefold |
| Black | Blackish |
| Sick | Sickly |

Formation of adjectives from nouns is more in number when compared to verbs and other adjectives.

## Exercises

**I. Form adjectives from the following nouns:**

1. ease ____________________
2. pity ____________________
3. time ____________________
4. heaven ____________________
5. room ____________________
6. peace ____________________
7. health ____________________
8. love ____________________
9. pomp ____________________
10. wood ____________________
11. sense ____________________
12. quarrel ____________________
13. hill ____________________
14. mountain ____________________
15. need ____________________
16. child ____________________
17. prince ____________________
18. progress ____________________
19. pain ____________________
20. doubt ____________________

**II. Use each of the adjectives in a sentence of your own:**

*Example:* Healthy–Swimming is a healthy exercise.

1. happy ______________________________
2. sad ______________________________
3. lazy ______________________________
4. big ______________________________
5. small ______________________________
6. soft ______________________________
7. harsh ______________________________
8. hard ______________________________
9. clever ______________________________
10. dull ______________________________
11. handsome ______________________________
12. certain ______________________________
13. strong ______________________________
14. quick ______________________________
15. cruel ______________________________
16. wise ______________________________
17. foolish ______________________________
18. rich ______________________________
19. poor ______________________________
20. young ______________________________

**III. Use as many suitable adjectives with each of the following Nouns:**

*Example:*

*Adjectives*

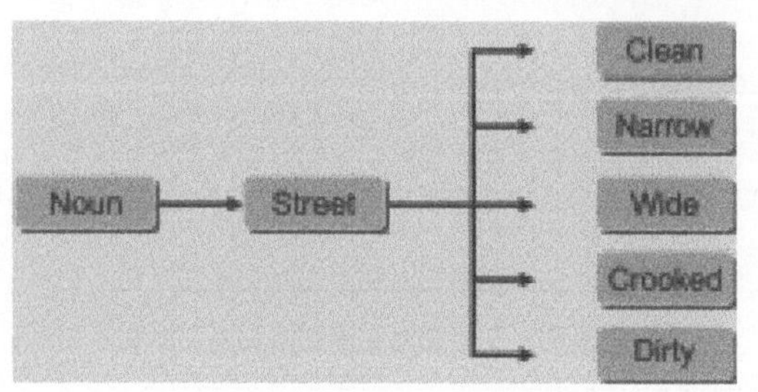


a clean street

a narrow street

a wide street

a crooked street

a dirty street

Man

Health

Progress

Room

Hospital

Cloth

Doctor

Janitor

**IV. Write the adjectives opposite in meaning to the following:**

| | | | |
|---|---|---|---|
| clean | ____________ | careful | ____________ |
| industrious | ____________ | experienced | ____________ |
| patient | ____________ | barren | ____________ |
| soft | ____________ | slow | ____________ |
| clear | ____________ | friendly | ____________ |
| wild | ____________ | beautiful | ____________ |
| lean | ____________ | honest | ____________ |
| strong | ____________ | | |

## Comparison of Adjectives

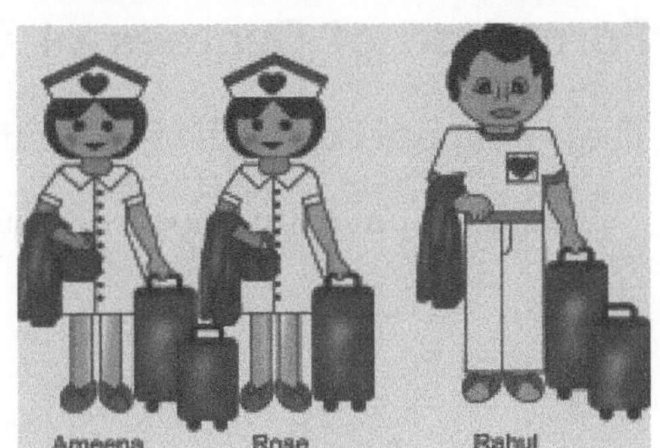


1. Nurse Rahul is clever.
2. Nurse Rose is cleverer than Rahul.
3. Nurse Ameena is the cleverest of them all.

In the first sentence, the adjective clever just tells us that nurse Rahul has the quality of being clever, without saying how much of this quality he has.

Thus, the adjective *clever* is said to be in the *Positive Degree.*

*Positive degree* of an adjective is the adjective in its simplest form. It is used when no comparison is made. It shows the existence of a quality which *we speak about*.

In the second sentence, the adjective cleverer tells us that nurse Rose when compared with nurse Rahul has more of the *quality* of being clever.

Thus, the adjective *cleverer* is said to be in the *Comparative Degree.*

*Comparative Degree* of an adjective shows a higher degree of the quality than the Positive, and it is used when two things are compared with each other.

In the third sentence, the adjective cleverest tells us that among the three nurses, nurse Ameena has the greatest amount of the quality of being clever.

Thus, the adjective *cleverest* is called the *Superlative Degree.*

Superlative degree of an adjective shows the *highest* degree of the quality, and is used when *more than two things are compared.*

This change in form of the adjectives (clever, cleverer, cleverest) to show comparison, is called as the three degrees of comparison.

***Remember***

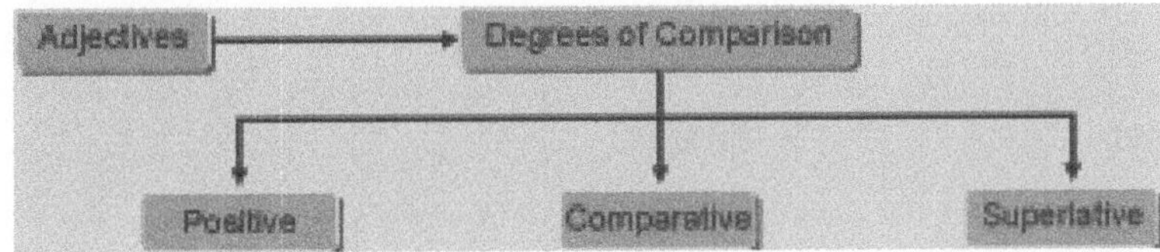

## Formation of Degrees of Comparison

The question arises do all the adjectives have degrees of comparison?

Yes. They have. But the formation differs from one adjective to another.

*Like–*

| ***Positive*** | ***Comparative*** | ***Superlative*** |
|---|---|---|
| Sweet | Sweeter | Sweetest |
| Good | Better | Best |
| Learned | More learned | Most learned |

One cannot say

| | | | |
|---|---|---|---|
| Good | Gooder | Goodest | × |
| Learned | Learneder | Learnedest | × |

Here are some ways in which the formation of comparative and superlative takes place.

**I. Most adjectives of *one* syllable and some of more than one, form the comparative and superlative degrees by adding -er and -est to the positive.**

*Example:*

| ***Positive*** | ***Comparative*** | ***Superlative*** |
|---|---|---|
| Sweet | Sweeter | Sweetest |
| Small | Smaller | Smallest |
| Tall | Taller | Tallest |
| Bold | Bolder | Boldest |

When the positive ends in 'e', only 'r' and 'st' are added respectively in comparative and superlative.
*Example:*

| | | |
|---|---|---|
| Brave | Braver | Bravest |
| Fine | Finer | Finest |
| White | Whiter | Whitest |

| | | |
|---|---|---|
| Pale | Paler | Palest |
| Large | Larger | Largest |

When the Positive ends in 'y', preceded by a consonant, 'y' is changed to 'i' before adding 'er' and 'est'.

| | | |
|---|---|---|
| Happy | Happier | Happiest |
| Easy | Easier | Easiest |
| Heavy | Heavier | Heaviest |
| Healthy | Healthier | Healthiest |
| Busy | Busier | Busiest |

When the positive is a word of one syllable and ends in a single consonant preceded by a short vowel, this consonant is doubled before adding 'er' and 'est'. Like–

| | | |
|---|---|---|
| Red | Redder | Reddest |
| Big | Bigger | Biggest |
| Hot | Hotter | Hottest |
| Fat | Fatter | Fattest |

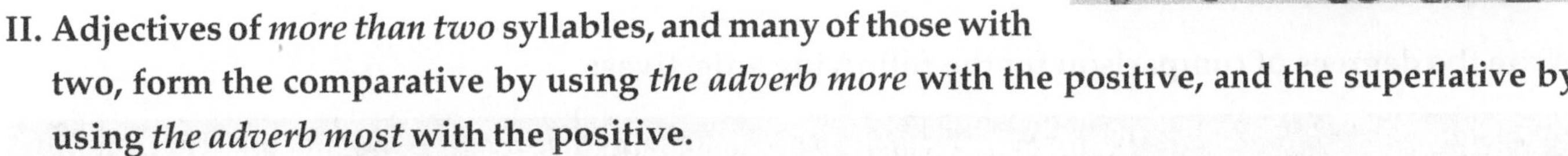

**II. Adjectives of *more than two* syllables, and many of those with two, form the comparative by using *the adverb more* with the positive, and the superlative by using *the adverb most* with the positive.**

***Example:***

| *Positive* | *Comparative* | *Superlative* |
|---|---|---|
| Beautiful | more beautiful | most beautiful |
| Difficult | more difficult | most difficult |
| Courageous | more courageous | most courageous |
| Learned | more learned | most learned |
| Proper | more proper | most proper |

**III. Irregular Comparison: Some adjectives are compared irregularly. Which means, their comparative and superlative are not formed from the positive. Like–**

| *Positive* | *Comparative* | *Superlative* |
|---|---|---|
| Good | Better | Best |
| Well | Better | Best |
| Bad | Worse | Worst |
| Evil | Worse | Worst |
| (There is no evil | eviller evillest) | |
| Ill | Worse | Worst |
| Little | Less/Lesser | Least |
| Much | More | Most (quantity) |
| Many | More | Most (number) |
| Late | Later/Latter | Latest/Last |
| Old | Older/Elder | Oldest/Eldest |
| Far | Farther | Farthest |



## Exercise

**Write the degrees of comparison for the following adjectives:**

| Sl. No. | Positive Degree | Comparative Degree | Superlative Degree |
|---|---|---|---|
| 1. | Black | | |
| 2. | Excellent | | |
| 3. | Ill | | |
| 4. | Gloomy | | |
| 5. | Mad | | |
| 6. | Safe | | |
| 7. | Bad | | |
| 8. | Unjust | | |
| 9. | Gay | | |
| 10. | Able | | |

*Contd...*

*Contd...*

| Sl. No. | Positive Degree | Comparative Degree | Superlative Degree |
|---|---|---|---|
| 11. | Dry | | |
| 12. | Timid | | |
| 13. | Ugly | | |
| 14. | True | | |
| 15. | Severe | | |
| 16. | Exact | | |
| 17. | Agreeable | | |
| 18. | Difficult | | |
| 19. | Little | | |
| 20. | Few | | |
| 21. | Numerous | | |
| 22. | Merry | | |

If you are able to form sentences of your own for each form of the degrees of comparison for these words no doubts will remain. You will have mastered this aspect of adjectives.

Now in III method of forming the degrees of comparison, we come across double forms of comparative and superlative of the adjectives. Here are some of the ways to use them.

Let us first take later, latter; latest, last

Here later and latest refer to time. Latter and last refer to position.

*For example:*

1. Sister Nora is *later* than I expected.
2. She has not heard the *latest* news.
3. The *latter* pages of the nursing dictionary are uninteresting.
4. The *last* chapter in community nursing is easy.
5. Abdul is the *last* patient in the general ward.

Next we shall take the adjectives elder, older; eldest, oldest.

Elder and eldest are used only for human beings.

Older and oldest are used for both human beings and things.

1. Dinesh is sister Nivedita's *elder* brother.
2. Dr Doshi is the *eldest* son of matron Sarika.
3. Enchey monastery is the *oldest* monastery I have seen.
4. Surgeon Mike is *older* than surgeon Avinash.

## Exercises

**I. Fill in the blank spaces with 'later' or 'latter':**

1. Most of the doctors accepted the __________ proposal.
2. The __________ part of the text-book shows signs of mishandling.
3. At a __________ date, he was placed in charge of the burns Ward.
4. Is there no __________ news than yesterday's?

**II. Fill in the blank spaces with 'older' or 'elder':**

1. I have an __________ brother.
2. Anita is __________ than Rita by five years.
3. Their __________ sister is in the Armed Forces Medical Corps.
4. He is the __________ of the two brothers.

**III. Fill in the blank spaces with 'eldest' or 'oldest':**

1. She is the __________ member of the Nursing College Committee.
2. Here comes Savitha, the Medical Officer's __________ daughter.
3. The __________ mosque in the city is near the bus station.
4. This is the __________ disease known to mankind.

**IV. Fill in the blank spaces with 'latest' or 'last':**

1. The __________ news from the operation theater is very disturbing.
2. The __________ time I saw her, she was very happy.
3. Today is the __________ day for submitting examination fees.
4. We expect to get the __________ news in a few minutes.

**V. Point out the adjectives and name the degree of comparison:**

1. The old nurse had seen better days.
2. Make less noise.
3. Hunger is the best sauce.
4. Her knife is sharper than yours.
5. She hopes the matter will be cleared up some day.
6. The nurse said, "I have other things to attend to."
7. No news is good news.
8. Dr Raman is taller than his father.
9. This stethoscope is longer than that stethoscope.
10. The clinical supervisor watched as the ward boys brought in the largest box into the laboratory.
11. The children's ward is always tidy.
12. This student nurse makes beds quicker than the other nurses.
13. Dr Rohan is the best surgeon in the Orthopaedic department.
14. The patient in ward 9 is stronger today.
15. This is the most complicated formula that I have learnt.

**VI. Supply the appropriate comparatives or superlatives given in the brackets:**

Malaria transmission does not occur at altitudes above 2000-2500 m, although in some parts of the world the ceiling is __________ (lower/lowest). Many high altitude regions of the world are situated in countries where there is a high risk of acute diarrhoeal illness in travellers. At __________ (less/least) 80 per cent of cases of travellers' diarrhoea have an infectious aetiology. In __________ (more/most) cases the pathogen is bacterial with enterotoxigenic *Escherichia coli* continuing to the __________ (more commonly/most commonly) encountered organism. Needless to say, avoiding the ingestion of enteropathogens is the __________ way (better/best) to prevent travellers'diarrhoea. After initiation of treatment, diarrhoea typically lasts about one day, whereas it lasts two or four days if untreated. As with antimicrobial chemoprophylaxis, quinolones are the __________ (more effective/most effective). The __________ (better/best) results have been achieved with the combination of an antimicrobial agent and the antimotility agent, loperamide in adults.

You will have noticed that when positive degree is used, the sentence structure is usually simple. When Comparative Degree is used 'than' is added after the adjective. When superlative degree is used, 'the' is always added before writing the adjective. Why is 'the' added is answered in the next topic Articles.

## Position of the Adjectives

Adjectives cannot be placed anywhere in a sentence. They have to be placed in a certain way. This is because their basic function is to describe a noun or verb.

There are two major positions of the adjectives.

1. Before a noun, and
2. After certain verbs

*Example:*

1. Before a noun:

i. The infected (Adjective) cotton (Noun) must be burnt.

ii. The arrogant (Adjective) Medical Administrator (Noun) pushed me away.

2. After verbs like seem, appear, look, sound, smell…

*Example:*

i. The doctor seems (Verb) quiet (Adjective) today.

ii. I felt (Verb) relieved (Adjective) when the doctor told my father was fine.

iii. Rajiv looks (Verb) tired (Adjective) at the end of the day.

## ARTICLES

Strictly speaking, there are only two articles. (Yes. You did read right. Don't get confused. Read on and you will know more.) They are 'a' and 'the'. Now 'a' undergoes a change before a word beginning with a vowel sound. (Remember vowel and consonants from Chapter 1). The change is 'an'. This is used before a word beginning with a vowel sound. Do not confuse yourself by adding 'an' before every word that starts with a vowel. Some words begin with a consonant, yet, have a vowel sound. Such words too have 'an' written before them. Let us know more about these articles.

The adjectives 'a' an', the' are called Articles. They are generally found in Demonstrative Adjectives.

There are two types of articles. They are:

1. Definite Article, and
2. Indefinite Article.



### 1. Definite Article

This article points out a particular person or thing. This is may be to show the person or thing to be unique or single out this person or thing.

'The' is the article which does this. Therefore it is called as a Definite Article.

*Example:* She saw the teacher (mean some particular teacher)

### 2. Indefinite Article

This article leaves 'indefinite' the person or thing spoken of. 'a' and 'an' do this. Therefore they are called as indefinite article.

*Example:* A nurse (means any nurse)

An apple (means any apple)

At this point you would ask the question, "Where do I use the, a, and an?"

It is easy once you understand the concept. So, here are some rules to be followed while using articles. Let us first begin the use of the definite article 'the'.

## Use of the Definite Article

'The' is used–

i. When a specific/particular person or thing is spoken of. Or, it is also used when we refer to a person or thing already referred to.

*Example:* *The* rice you asked for is over.

*The* boy in the last row, with *the* red pencil is naughty.

Let us go *to the* movie.

ii. When a singular noun is meant to represent a whole class.

*Example:* *The* cat loves fish.

*The* camel is a beautiful animal.

*The* dogs bark and wag their tail.

iii. When names of gulfs, rivers, seas, oceans, islands and mountain-ranges are referred to.

*Example:* *The* Gulf of Kutch.

*The* Brahmaputra flows swiftly.

*The* Indian Ocean can be seen at Kanyakumari.

*The* Galapagos Islands are famous for their flora and fauna.

The Kanchendzonga is *the* only mountain peak to be featured on a currency note.

iv. Before the names of holy books.

*Example:* *The* Mahabharatha

*The* Bible

*The* Koran

*The* Zend-Avesta

v. Before common nouns that are names of things unique to their kind or type.

*Example:* *The* sun,

*The* sky

*The* moon

vi. Before a proper noun only when it is qualified by an adjective or a defining adjectival clause.

*Example:* *The* immortal Wordsworth.

*The* Mrs. Jagannath whom you met this morning is my mother.

vii. With ordinals.(Remember the chapter Nouns—you have ordinals , that is the depicting of numbers by their order in words.)

*Example:* She was *the* first patient to enter the clinic.

The twentieth chapter is interesting.

viii. With superlatives (remember Adjectives—Degrees of Comparison).

*Example:* *The* mightiest of warriors have a weak point.

This is *the* best class in child care.

***Note:*** 'the' is never used with positive and comparative degrees.

ix. Before musical instruments.

*Example:* She can play *the* sitar well.

He is learning to play *the* piano.

[Generally people use—He is learning piano. This is wrong. None can learn an instrument all by itself. One can only learn to play any instrument.]

x. Before an adjective when the noun is understood.

*Example:* *The* **elite** are always welcomed everywhere. (rich people)

xi. As an adverb with comparitives.

*Example:* *The* more *the* merrier.

xii. Before the names of universities, colleges and ranks.

*Example:* The University of Mysore.

The National College

The Principal

[NOTE: Mysore University is right too. But when we write or speak this way 'the' and 'of' are omitted]

## Omission of 'the'

1. **Usually 'the' is not used before plural nouns.**

   *Example:* I like skirts and trousers.

   Students try to study till the last minute before an exam begins.

> ***Note:*** If the nouns are specified, 'the' must be used.

*Example:* She loves chocolates but *the* chocolates of that brand are bitter.

*The* young nurses who work in remote villages must be admired for their commitment.



2. **'The' is not used before proper nouns.**

   *Example:* Shanta is a doctor.

   Asia is developing quickly.

3 **`The' is omitted before names of relations like father, mother, aunt, uncle.**

*Example:* Father went to Kolkata.

Aunt left all her money to me.

> ***Note:*** 1. Here My father, my aunt is understood. It is not written.
>
> 2. When the same names of relatives are used in a general context, depending on the sentence, 'the' is used.

*Example:* *The* mothers were angry when the school cancelled the holidays.

All *the* fathers agreed to talk to the coach.

4. 'the' is not used to denote the position that is normally held by one person at a given time.

   *Example:* Mr.Yogesh became principal of the college in 2004.

   She was elected chairperson of the Board.

## Use of the Indefinite Article 'a'

This is used to

1. to denote the original numerical sense of *one*.

   *Example:* Twelve inches make *a* foot.

   None said *a* word.

   *A* bird in the hand is worth two in the bush.

2. to show 'a particular' person in a vague sense.

   *Example:* *A* Tom Cunha is suspected by the police (a certain person named Tom Cunha).

   One evening *a* student knocked on the professor's door.

3. to give the sense of any, to single out an individual as a representative of a group.

   *Example:* *A* student should study well.

   *A* camel is a useful animal.



## Use of 'an'

'An' is used only before a word that has a vowel sound. The sound of the initial letter and not the letter itself that decides whether we use 'a' or 'an' before it.

| *Example:* | a pen | an ice-cream |
|---|---|---|
| | a book | an orange |
| | a university | an umbrella |
| | a European | an Eskimo |

Don't get confused here. Both 'university' and 'umbrella' begin with the vowel 'u'. But, only 'umbrella' has the vowel sound. Similarly, European has a consonant sound (you). The 'e' in Eskimo has a vowel sound (e) whereas 'e' in European has a consonant sound (you).

## Complete Absence of Articles

**No article is used–**

1. Before proper nouns.

   *Example:* She went to Scotland and met her friend Sheila.

2. Before abstract noun used in a general sense.

   *Example:* Honesty is the best policy.

   Cricket is popular in India.

   Many students find mathematics tough to learn.

   [Here honesty, cricket and mathematics are abstract nouns. For clarification on abstract nouns see the chapter Nouns]

3. Before languages.

   *Example:* We are studying English.

   They like Spanish.

4. Before uncountable nouns. Like–

   Water is essential for life.

   Blood is red in colour

   Rice is the staple diet in India.

   [water, blood and rice are uncountable nouns]

5. Before the names of the most diseases and illness.

   *Example:* Tuberculosis killed many in the early twentieth century.

   Viral fever is rampant during monsoon.

> *Note:* I have a headache / She has the swine flue } Articles are used here to specify

6. Before nouns like 'school, college, church, bed, table, hospital, market, prison when they are visited for their primary purposes.

   *Example:* I learnt Hindi at school.

   They go to church on Sundays.

   'He stays in bed till ten every Sunday.'

   My grandfather is still in hospital.

> ***Note:*** The above mentioned nouns when used as a place to visit have suitable articles placed before them.

   *Example:* The school is near my home.

   Roger met me in the church.

   The bed is very musty and old.

   I went to the hospital to see a doctor.

7. Before names of materials. Like, Gold is an attractive metal.

   Cotton grows in India, America and Egypt.



## Exercises

**I. Fill up the blanks with 'a', 'an', 'the' where necessary. Write × if no article is required.**

1. ________copper is ________useful metal.
2. Dolores works in ________shop selling gramophone records.
3. "I want ________record. One I heard on ________radio this morning," She said.
4. Did you say she was going to ________Oxford, or ________Cambridge?
5. Mind crossing ________street, won't you?
6. ________wrist watch had been given to her only two months ago.
7. She is ________cleverest girl in ________class.

8. ________first singer was more pleasing than________second.
9. They had to walk half ________mile across the fields.
10. She grew worse, and I had to call ________doctor.
11. ________low, swampy land south of Florida's Lake Okeechobee teems with exotic subtropical wildlife ________naturalist's paradise.
12. Honest people speak ________truth.
13. Do you see ________black board?
14. The world is ________happy place.
15. They returned after ________hour.
16. I first met her ________year ago.
17. Varanasi and Jerusalem are ________holy cities.
18. You are ________fool to say that.
19. Nurse Anita has come without ________umberalla.
20. He is ________untidy boy.



**II. Insert Articles where necessary.**

1. Sun sets in west.
2. The soldier lost eye in battle.
3. I like to exercise in open air.
4. Eskimos build houses of snow and ice.
5. Draw map of India.
6. What beautiful scene this is!
7. National Malaria Control Programme was launched in 1953 to reduce incidence of malaria.
8. Diabetic patient mostly feels very thirsty and hungry and passes frequent and excessive urine.
9. Coronary Heart Disease is one of commonest causes of death in countries with high standard of living.

10. Blood groups are based on presence or absence of certain antigens on surfaces of RBC and of certain antibodies in blood plasma.
11. Mountain climbers with head injuries should be evacuated (air lifted) as rapidly as possible.
12. In unconscious patient collar should remain *in situ* during evacuation.
13. Patient needs to sleep for 6 hours before going for operation.
14. Special pass is needed to enter ICU.
15. Every morning student nurses sponge bedridden patients.
16. It was proudest moment of his life.
17. Bold eagle is national bird of USA.
18. Andamans are group of islands in Bay of Bengal.
19. Arian is dynamic.
20. As intelligent as owl.

**III. Insert 'the' where necessary in the passage below.**

Himalayan giants are notoriously reclusive and most are remote and distant Khangchendzonga, however, is much more flamboyant. Sikkim Himalayas, where Himalayan layers of Siwaliks, Lower Himalayan Range and Great Himalayas, all collide into one compact upheaval of mountainscape, throws up Khangchendzonga its position as third highest mountain in world. Mountain, however, lowers its defenses only for those wishing to mediate on its visage; for climbers, even striking base camp is not easily achieved. Khangchendzonga is temperamental and despite its accessibility, it is feared in mountaineering circles as most difficult mountain. It remains to this day, most formidable antagonist.

Mountaineering equipment and skills have developed much since mountain was first attempted. But, no technology, no conditioning can prepare a person to remain stuck in their tents for 36 hours at a stretch at 7,400 metres while storm ranges outside. Two climbers, one a German and another Austrian experienced this while attempting mountain in April-May 2005 on 15th anniversary of first ascent. With temperature plunging to 20°C below zero inside tent, storm was forcing snow inside tent through breathing slits, humidity was high and high velocity winds outside collided with synthetic fibres of their tents to spark off miniature lightning displays zigzagging across the tents. They spent 36 excruciating hours getting battered by snow and ice and knowing all along that eventual push to summit, if it was at all allowed by weather, would demand hands-on rock climbing is a discomfiting thought that can disorient most seasoned of climbers. That is what this great mountain Khangchendzonga is all about, a mind-numbing assortment of contrasting challenges.

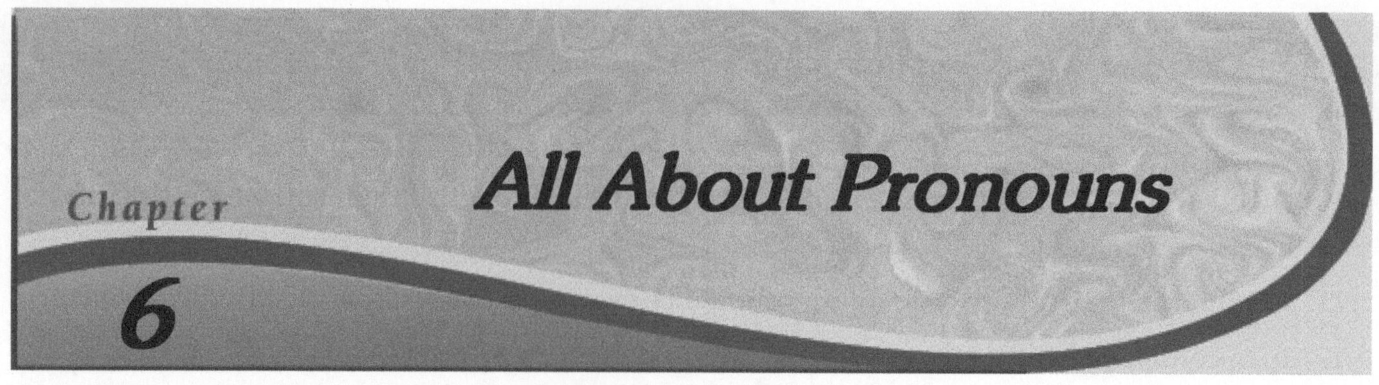


Definition: A word that is used instead of a noun is called a **Pronoun**.

*Example:* Paul Cherian is ill because Paul Cherian ate an ice-cream in cold weather.

Instead of repeating the proper noun (name of a person) we use he. The sentence becomes–

Paul Cherian is ill, because *he* ate an ice-cream in cold weather.

Look at these sentences:

| | |
|---|---|
| *I* am tall. | *We* are tall. |
| *He* is old. | *You* are stubborn. |
| *She* is nice. | *They* are nice. |
| *It* is ill. | |

I, we, he, you, she, they, it, are all pronouns.

Just as in the other parts of speech, we find different types of pronouns.

They are:

i. Personal Pronouns
ii. Reflexive and Emphatic Pronouns
iii. Indefinite Pronouns
iv. Relative Pronouns

We will briefly touch on all these types and not go into details. This is done to help you in understanding Pronouns. Once you learn and understand their usage, you can refer many Grammar books for your pleasure.

i. *Personal Pronouns:* In the above sentences, I, we, he, you, they, it, are called Personal Pronouns. This is so, as they stand for the three persons.

# All About Pronouns

1. The person speaking → also referred to as First Person.
2. The person spoken to → also referred to as Second Person, and
3. The person spoken of → also referred to as the Third Person.

## Different Forms of the Personal Pronouns

In these pronouns we have both the singular and plural forms.

| Sl. No. | First Person | (These are used for both Masculine and Feminine) | | | |
|---|---|---|---|---|---|
| 1. | First Person | *Singular* | *Plural* | | |
| | Nominative Case | I | We | | |
| | Possessive Case | my, mine | our, ours | | |
| | | Me | us | | |
| 2. | Second Person | (These too are used for both Masculine and Feminine.) | | | |
| | | *Singular* | *Plural* | | |
| | Nominative case | you | you | | |
| | Possessive case | your | your, yours | | |
| 3. | Third Person | (This has all three genders–Masculine, Feminine, and Neuter.) | | | |
| | | *Singular* | | | *Plural* |
| | | Masculine | Feminine | Neuter | All Genders |
| | Nominative case | he | she | it | they |
| | Possessive case | his | her, hers | its | their, theirs |
| | | him | her | it | them |

Here are some example sentences:

i. *I* have a lot of books.

ii. *We* went to the emergency ward together.

iii. *My* nursing notes are misplaced.

iv. Those needles are *mine*.

v. Suby Thomas is *our* teacher in English.

vi. These bedclothes are *ours.*

vii. "It's *me* who wrote on the wall", said the child.

viii. He is going to church with *us.*

ix. *You* are very untidy.

x. *Your* bag is torn.

xi. *Yours* is the first name in the register.

xii. The *ambulance driver* drove the ambulance fast. *He* drove the ambulance fast.

xiii. The staff nurses are working hard for the exams.

*They* are working hard for their exams

xiv. *She* was kind to all terminally ill patients.

xv. *The infection* / viral fever is contagious.

*It* is contagious.

xvi. Most of the orthopaedic operations are carried out by Dr Princy. *His* students are lucky to study under *him.*

xvii. *Her* mother is very understanding.

xviii. *Hers* is a tough job.

xix. *Their* mothers were waiting to talk to the teacher.

xx. The matron found the two naughty children outside the ward. *She* has brought *them* back to the ward.

In the above sentences you will notice that the possessive cases my, our, your, her, their, are called as possessive adjective, as they are used with nouns and do the work of adjectives.

*Example:*

1. That is *my* bag.
2. These are *your* notes.
3. This is *her* stethoscope.

> ***Note # 1:*** The word *his* is used both as an Adjective and as a Pronoun.
> *Example:*
> 1. This is *his* thermometer. (Possessive Adjective)
> 2. This radiology book is *his*. (Possessive Pronoun)

At this point you will notice that a pronoun can be used at any point in the sentence. It may be at the beginning, in the middle, or at the end of the sentence. This means they can be used as the subject or as the object in a sentence.

*Note # 2:* The various uses of the pronoun *it*:

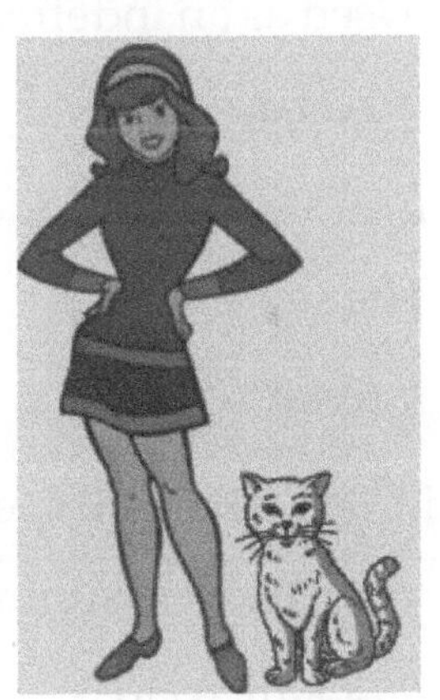

i. For inanimate things (things without life)

*Example:*

Here is your *Petridish*; take *it* away.

ii. For animals, unless the gender is specified when we speak.

*Example:*

She loves her cat and cannot do without *it*.

The cow fell and broke *its* leg.

iii. To refer to a child, unless we wish to refer to the sex.

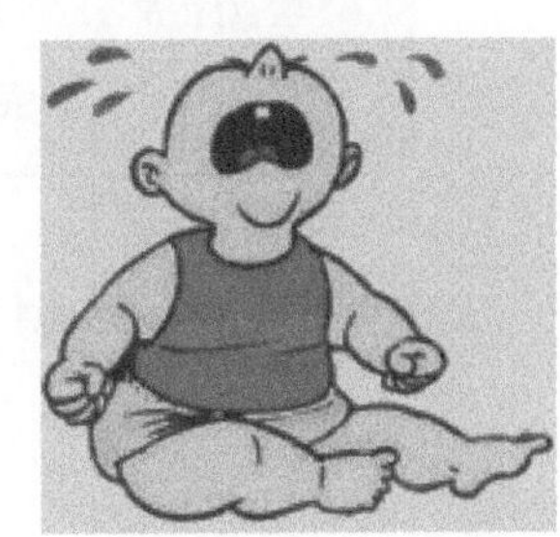

*Example:*

When nurse Ramesh saw the child, *it* was howling in pain.

This baby has torn *its* clothes.

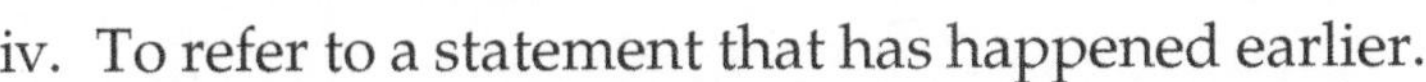

iv. To refer to a statement that has happened earlier.

*Example:*

She is telling a lie; and she knows *it*.

v. Used as a temporary subject before the verb to be when the real subject follows.

*Example:*

*It* is easy to find fault (To find fault is easy.)

*It* is doubtful whether they will write the exam.

vi. To stress the importance of the noun or pronoun.

*Example:*

*It* was you who shouted loudly in the corridor.

*It* was nurse Reji who first said no.

vii. Used as an indefinite of an Impersonal Verb.

*Example:*

*It* snows, here *it* does not stand for any noun, but the verb can supply the noun as The snow snows.

*It* roars

viii. Used when we speak of the time or the weather.

*Example: It* is sunny.

*It* is eight o'clock.

> ***Note # 3:*** When two or more Singular Nouns are joined by and, the Pronoun used for them must be Plural.

*Example:* Paul and Stalin are good doctors. *They* are trusted by their patients.

> ***Note # 4:*** It is good manners to say–

'You and I' not 'I and you'

'You and He' not 'He and you'

'Harry and I' not 'I and Harry'

'She/He and I' not 'I and she/he'

> *Note # 5:*
> 1. I is called first person singular pronoun
>    It refers to oneself in speech or in writing.
> 2. *You* is used both in singular and plural.

## Exercises

**I. Identify the correct forms of personal pronouns and fill in the blanks:**

i. Doctors ___________

ii. Matron Mini ___________

iii. Head nurse Mathew ________

iv. Bag ________

v. Conical flask_____________

vi. Pillow____________

vii. The sutures___________

viii. Dr Nabeela and Dr Rai_________

ix. Ibuprofen tablets___________

x. Antibiotics______________

**II. Fill in the blanks with the correct pronouns:**

i. "____ wish ____ hadn't laughed so much", said Alice.

ii. Scarlet, ______ are an untidy girl.

iii. The female tiger is called a tigress. ____ has no name.

iv. The male nurse is reading the blood report of the elderly patient. _____looks satisfied.

v. Camel is called as the beast of burden. _____is used to carry goods across the desert.

vi. Her sisters are going for scanning today. _____are very anxious about the results.

vii. My friend and I do yoga everyday. _____want to have good health.

viii. All birds do not build _____ nests in trees.

ix. Sadhana lost _____ medical kit bag yesterday.

x. Nurse Suresh and nurse Ramesh are good friends and good nurses. _______ is a good team.

xi. ______ tough to study all the chapters just before the exams. ________must study ______ from the beginning of the term.

xii. The head nurse praised ______ for maintaining clean wards.

xiii. ______ socks are too tight.

xiv. "That is _____. Mine is here", said Ruby showing two piles of books.

xv. Karim found ______ horse in a meadow this morning.

xvi. ______ pen writes better.



Let us now look into Reflexive and Emphatic Pronouns.

## Reflexive and Emphatic Pronouns

If -self is added to my, your, him, her, it, and

-selves is added to our, your, them, we get compound personal pronouns.

i.e., myself, yourself, ourselves, yourselves

singular in usage plural in usage.

When an action done by the subject turns back (reflects) upon the subject, such pronouns are called Reflexive Pronouns.

*Example:*

1. He hurt *himself*. They hurt themselves.
2. I went to the department myself. We hit ourselves.
3. He had a fractured leg. Yet, he climbed the stairs all by himself.
4. The cow hurt itself.

**Emphatic Pronouns** are the compound personal pronouns that are used for the sake of emphasis.

*Example:*

1. I will do it *myself.*
2. They saw the Queen *herself.*
3. The village *itself* is not very large.
4. They *themselves* admitted their mistake.

For ease of remembering different pronouns and their functions, here is a table.

| Person | Number | Subject | Object | Possessive | | Reflexive |
|---|---|---|---|---|---|---|
| | | | | Adjectival | Nominal | |
| First | Singular | I | me | my | mine | myself |
| | Plural | We | us | our | ours | ourselves |
| Second | Singular | You | you | Your | yours | yourself |
| | Plural | you | you | your | yours | yourselves |
| Third | Singular: | | | | | |
| | Masculine | he | him | his | his | himself |
| | Feminine | she | her | her | hers | herself |
| | Neuter | it | it | its | | itself |
| | Plural | they | them | their | theirs | themselves |

## Exercise

**Identify the reflexive pronouns and emphatic pronouns in these sentences:**

i. He will go himself.

ii. The nurse went to the nursing station, as he had cut himself while cleaning the scalpels.

iii. You express yourself perfectly.

iv. We wash ourselves when we get up.

| Reflexive Pronouns | Emphatic Pronouns |
|---|---|
| | |
| | |
| | |
| | |

| | Reflexive Pronouns | Emphatic Pronouns |
|---|---|---|
| v. The girls hid themselves. | | |
| vi. She has got herself into a mess. | | |
| vii. Cleopatra poisoned herself. | | |
| viii. He loved himself so much that he thought of no one else. | | |
| ix. Roshan tried to medicate himself. | | |
| x. I myself will speak to him. | | |
| xi. We gave ourselves a lot of trouble. | | |
| xii. Some depressed patients hate themselves. | | |
| xiii. She set herself an easy task. | | |
| xiv. The horse choked itself. | | |
| xv. Once the beep of the pulse oximeter stopped, the doctors stopped giving the cardiac pulmonary resuscitation themselves. | | |
| xvi. We rarely see ourselves as others see us. | | |
| xvii. The junior nurse had to clean all the bed - pans herself/ himself. | | |
| xviii. The orphaned boy had to go for the blood test all by himself. | | |
| xix. Lokesh and Peter tried to medicate their cold themselves. | | |
| xx. The electric car runs itself on batteries. | | |



## Indefinite Pronouns

*Definition:* Pronouns which refer to persons or things in a general way, and not to any person or thing in particular are called as **Indefinite Pronouns.**

*Example:*

i. *None* knew what to do.

*ii.* *One* cannot be too careful of *one's* good name.

*iii.* *All* were dead.

*iv.* *Some* are born rich.

*v.* *Some* say he is a thief.

*vi.* *Somebody* ate all the food.

*vii.* *Nobody* was around to rescue the old man.

*viii.* *Few* escaped with minor injuries.

*ix.* *Many* of them were Hindus.

*x.* We did not see *any* of them again.

*xi.* Do good to *others*.

*xii.* *Everybody's* business is nobody's business.

*xiii.* Most of these are also used as adjectives.

| Indefinite Pronouns | Adjectives |
|---|---|
| *Few* escaped unhurt. | She is a woman of *few* words. |
| *Some* drink milk thrice a day. | *Some* milk was spilt. |
| *One* must not praise oneself. | I will take you there *one* day. |

***Note # 1:*** When anybody, everybody, everyone, anyone, each are used, the pronoun he or she is used according to the context.

*Example:* I shall be happy to help *everyone* of my girls in *her* studies.

***Note # 2:*** When sex is not determined, the pronoun of the masculine gender is used. This is, because, there is no singular pronoun of the third person to represent both the male and female.

*Example:* *Everyone* likes to have *his* way.

Each must do *his* best.

## Relative Pronouns

Read the pairs of sentences below.

i. I met nurse Linda. Linda had just returned from her class.

ii. She has found the syringe. She had lost the syringe.

iii. Here are the notes. You lent me the notes.

Now let us combine each of the above pairs into one sentence.

i. I met nurse Linda who had just returned from her class.

ii. She has found the syringe which she lost.

iii. Here are the notes that you lent me.



What is the work done by each of the words *who, which,* and *that*?

Let us examine it.

In the first sentence, the word 'who' is used instead of Linda. Therefore, 'who' does the work of a Pronoun. This word also joins or connects two statements. Therefore it does the work of a conjunction. So, the word 'who' does double work—the work of a pronoun and also that of a conjunction.

Therefore we can call it a conjunctive pronoun. But, it refers or relates to the noun Linda. So it is called a Relative Pronoun.

Now you show how `which' and `that' are relative pronouns

______________________________________________

______________________________________________

______________________________________________

______________________________________________

______________________________________________

______________________________________________

## Use of Relative Pronouns

1. 'Who 'is generally used for *persons* only. It may refer to either a Singular Noun or a Plural Noun.

*Example:*

i. He *who* hesitates is lost.

ii. The doctor *who* is honest is trusted by his patients.

2. 'Whose' is used in speaking about persons. Sometimes it is used for things without life .

*Example:*

The sun *whose* rays give life to the earth, was regarded as God by ancient civilizations.

3. 'Which' is used for inanimate objects as well as for animals. It may refer to either a Singular Noun or a plural noun.

*Example:*

i. The time *which* is lost is lost forever.

ii. The dog *which* I sold is a labrador.

4. 'That' is used for persons and things. It may refer to either a singular noun or a plural noun.

*Example:*

i. Take anything *that* you like.

ii. This is the doctor *that* I told you of.

iii. I have lost the pen *that* you gave me.

iv. She was the most eloquent speaker *that* I ever heard.

5. 'That' is also used after who, what.

*Example:*

Who am I *that* I should object.

6. 'What' is used for things only.

*Example:*

i. *What* cannot be cured must be endured.

ii. She means *what* she says.

iii. They found *what* they were looking for.

## Exercises

**I. Fill in the blanks with suitable relative pronouns:**

i. We like children ___________ speak the truth.

ii. She knows you __________ you mean.

iii. She has gone to Thailand __________ is her birth place.

iv. Where is the beaker __________ I gave you?

v. Is this the road _________ leads to the hospital?

vi. Listen to __________ the professor says.

vii. Bronchitis is an inflammation of the mucous membrane _________ causes the affected person to cough.

viii. Bulimia is a disease ________ affects young girls.

ix. A sense organ or sensory nerve ending ________ is stimulated by and reacts to certain chemical stimuli is called chemoreceptor.

x. No one can lose _____ they never had.

xi. Did you receive the package ________ I sent last week?

xii. One ______ is a practitioner of some kind of therapy is called a therapist.

**II. Combine the following pairs of sentences by using a relative pronoun (who/that/which):**

i. A boy was injured in the accident. He is now in hospital.

_______________________________________________

ii. The nurse answered the phone in the nursing station. He told me you were away.

_______________________________________________

_______________________________________________

iii. A waiter served us. He was very impolite and impatient.

_______________________________________________

iv. A hospital was destroyed in the tsunami. It has now been rebuilt.

_______________________________________________

v. A bus goes to the airport. It runs every half hour.

______________________________________________

vi. I heard a song. The song pleased me.

______________________________________________

vii. I know a boy. The boy has a wooden leg.

______________________________________________

viii. I know a man. The man has been to Antarctica.

______________________________________________

ix. Here is the doctor. The doctor cured me of rheumatic fever.

______________________________________________

x. Meet nurse Asha. Nurse Asha looked after Aliya in the ICU.

______________________________________________



**III. In this exercise, you have to explain what some words mean. Choose the right meaning from the box and then write a sentence with *Who*.**

| | |
|---|---|
| He/she | steals from a shop.<br>does't believe in God.<br>teaches children in school.<br>scientist who studies anatomy.<br>designs interiors of a building.<br>a doctor trained to perform surgery. |
| He/she | prepare and sell medicines.<br>person works with you.<br>doctor treating the medical conditions and diseases of women.<br>doctor studying blood and its diseases.<br>cuts, washes and shapes hair. |

**Some words are given below (1-10) and meaning of each word has been explained in the box above. Make a sentence with the meaning from the box and write in the blank space given opposite each of the words.**

## Example

(an interior decorator) An interior decorator is someone who decorates interiors of a building.

1. (an anatomist) ____________________
2. (a shoplifter) ____________________
3. (an atheist) ____________________
4. (a chemist) ____________________
5. (a colleague) ____________________
6. (a teacher) ____________________
7. (a surgeon) ____________________
8. (a gynecologist) ____________________
9. (a hematologist) ____________________
10. (a hair-stylist) ____________________



**Choose the correct possessive pronouns or possessive adjectives and fill in the blanks:**

i. The surgeon is examining__________ infected eye.

(a) my (c) I

(b) mine (d) None of the above.

ii. The chemist gave __________ medicines and not __________ medicines.

(a) you, he (c) your and his

(b) your, he (d) you and your

iii. The university will announce __________ results tomorrow.

(a) we (c) ours

(b) them (d) our.

iv. __________ hemoglobin count is within normal limits.

(a) It (c) Her

(b) Me (d) They

v. The student nurses are admiring _________ brand new books.

(a) their (c) his

(b) her (d) them

vi. The neurologist spoke calmly to _________ patients.

(a) them (c) my

(b) his (d) none of the above.

vii. _______ six-year-old son opens _______ bowel once every two days.

(a) His, his (c) His, her

(b) Her, her (d) My, mine.

Chapter 7

# All About Verbs

Look at these sentences:

Shahid *sings.*

The bell *rings.*

Anuradha is *praised.*

Shyam is *promoted.*

The door *is* new.

I *feel* happy.

Paper *is* thin.

The words in *italics* tell us something about a person or thing. These tell us what a person or thing does as in the first two sentences. In the next two sentences the words in italics tell us what is done to a person or thing. In the last three sentences italicized words tell us what a person or thing is.

In other words, the above said words show an action (state of being) of a person or object. Such words are called as verbs.

## Definition

A verb is a word used to denote action (state of being) about a person or thing.

Often Verbs consist of more than one word. Like,

The boys *were playing* football.

She *has learnt* German.

The phone *had been ringing.*

## Exercise

**Identify the verbs in the following sentences:**

1. The crow flew down and stole the coconut.
2. The bus was driven rashly.
3. New brooms sweep clean.
4. The boy was waiting for the bell.
5. The students wrote the exam.
6. I was singing in the shower.
7. Dr Rao gave the injection to the child.
8. Nurse Amritha is talking to the little boy in bed 7.
9. Consultants are expensive to hire.
10. The architect designed this building.

Observe the following sentences:

1. Nurse Nora *is inserting* the catheter into the hand.
2. The child *laughs* softly.

In sentence 1, the action denoted by the verb *inserts passes over* from the doer or subject Nora to some object hand. Such a verb (*inserts*) is called as a transitive verb (Transitive means Passing over).

In sentence 2, the action denoted by the verb *laughs* stops with the doer or subject child and *does not pass over* to an object. Such a verb is called as an intransitive verb (intransitive means not passing over).

## Definition

A verb that denotes an action which *passes over* from the doer or subject to an object is called a transitive verb.

## Definition

A verb that denotes an action which *does not pass over* or which expresses a state of being is called an intransitive verb.

Sometimes a transitive verb can be used as an intransitive verb. Like,

| Transitive | Intransitive |
|---|---|
| 1. The patient *fought* the disease. | 1. Some boys *fight* very fiercely. |
| 2. The blast *sank* the submarine. | 2. The submarine *sank* quickly. |
| 3. "*Ring* the bell dear", said Matilda. | 3. The siren *rang* loudly. |
| 4. The chauffer *stopped* the car. | 4. The car *stopped* suddenly. |
| 5. She *speaks* the truth. | 5. She *spoke* softly. |

***Note:*** Some verbs like *come, go, fall, die, sleep,* and *lie* denote actions which cannot ***be done*** to anything. Therefore, they cannot be used transitively.



## Exercise

**Underline the verbs in the following sentences and identify whether it is a transitive or intransitive verb.**

1. The moon shines brightly.
2. The man cut his hand with a knife.
3. The power was cut this morning.
4. The sun sets in the west.
5. The nursing station is busy the entire day.
6. I looked out from the balcony.
7. The dog walks.
8. The boys ran down the street.
9. Many trees fell in the monsoon.
10. Rahul flew his kite.
11. The donkey kicked the man.
12. How do you feel?
13. He felt a severe pain in his stomach.

14. The bubble burst.
15. Please keep quiet.
16. I forgot his name.
17. The judge acquitted him of the charges against him.
18. Their talk does not interest me.
19. They speak too loudly.
20. She took shelter under a tree.

## ACTIVE AND PASSIVE VOICE

Now we come to an interesting topic in verbs. This is called Active and Passive Voice. Most of the times when we talk we use passive voice. "What is this?", you may ask. This tells us who is doing what. Yes, this sounds strange. Let us look into this now.

Look at the following sentences:

1. Shadab helps Sohan.
2. Sohan is helped by Shadab.

The above sentences express the same meaning. But in sentence 1, the form of the verb shows that the person (denoted by the subject) does *something.*

Shadab [(the person denoted by the subject) does something that is *help*]

Here the verb *helps* is said to be in the **Active Voice.**

In sentence 2, the form of the verb shows that *something* is done to the person denoted by the subject.

Something is *done* to Sohan (The person denoted by the subject).

Here the verb *helped* is said to be in **Passive Voice.**

In other words;

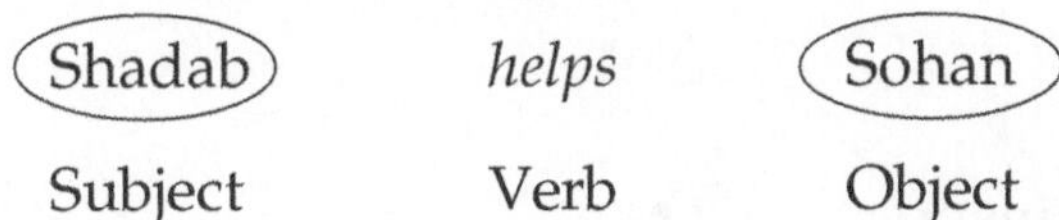


This is in Active Voice as the subject does something to the object.

| Sohan | *is helped by* | Shadab |
|---|---|---|
| Subject | Verb | Object |

Here the object of the previous sentence becomes the subject here and the subject of the previous sentence becomes the object in this sentence. This is in passive voice as something is done to [helped by] the subject by the object.

## Definition

Voice is the form of a verb which shows whether what is denoted by the subject does something or has something done to.

Here are some examples to show the change from the Active Voice to the Passive Voice.

| Active Voice | Passive Voice |
|---|---|
| 1. Mother *loves* Savitha. | 1. Savitha is *loved* by mother. |
| 2. The architect *is designing* the house. | 2. The house *is being* designed by the architect. |
| 3. The watchman *opened* the gate. | 3. The gate *was opened* by the watchman. |
| 4. Some nurses *were helping* the wounded children. | 4. The wounded children *were being helped* by some nurses. |
| 5. Who *did* this? | 5. By whom *was* this done? |
| 6. Why *did* your cousin paint such a poster? | 6. Why *was* such a poster painted by your cousin? |

You will notice that when the verb is changed from the active voice to the passive voice, the *object* of the transitive verb in the Active Voice becomes the *subject* of the verb in the passive voice.

Since the object of a verb in the active voice becomes the subject of the passive form, it is evident that *only transitive verbs can be used in the passive voice*, because an intransitive verb has no object.

The question now arises, **when is Active Voice used?**

It is used when the doer of an action is to be made prominent.

Sometimes the Active Voice involves the use of an indefinite or vague pronoun or nourn like somebody, they, people, we, someone, etc. as the subject. In such cases the Passive is generally preferred. Like,

i. Somebody has stolen my bag – Active voice (use of vague term)

My bag has been stolen – Passive voice (generally preferred)

ii. They asked me my name - Active voice

I was asked my name – Passive voice

iii. People speak English all over the world - Active voice

English is spoken all over the world- Passive voice

iv. Someone has invited me to the rock show - Active voice

I have been invited to the rock show – Passive voice

Have you noticed something in the above passive sentences?

Yes. The use of the agent 'by' is missing in the conversation from the active voice to the passive voice.

> ***Note:*** The *'by'* phrase cannot be avoided where the agent has some importance and is necessary to complete the sense.

## Exercise

**I. Identify the verbs [transitive or intransitive] in the following sentences and tell whether they are in the active voice or in the passive voice.**

1. The lioness killed the deer.

   Verb:_________ Voice:_____________

2. They compelled the children to eat bread.

   Verb:_________ Voice:_____________

3. The girl was bitten by a snake.

   Verb:_________ Voice:_____________

4. The spy was caught.

   Verb: _________ Voice: _____________

5. Srikanth made a kite.

   Verb:_________ Voice:_____________

6. The bus was burned.

   Verb:_________ Voice:_____________

7. The young man made a disturbance at the meeting.

   Verb:_________ Voice:_____________

8. The bird was killed by a cruel man.

   Verb:_________ Voice:_____________

9. The sudden noise frightened the cows.

   Verb:_________ Voice:_____________

10. She is loved by all.

    Verb:_________ Voice:_____________

11. The General's command was promptly obeyed.

    Verb:_________ Voice:_____________

12. Nothing will be gained by hurry.

    Verb: _________ Voice: _____________

13. The bird ate all the seeds.

    Verb: _________ Voice: _____________

14. They guarded the sheep.

    Verb: _________ Voice: _____________

15. This e-mail was sent last night.

    Verb: _________ Voice: _____________

**II. Change the following sentences from the active voice to the passive voice.**

1. The boy killed the mosquito.

_______________

2. Rajeev cut down the tree.

_______________

3. Joseph Black discovered carbon dioxide.

_______________

4. My teacher praised me.

_______________

5. Varun was making a kite.

_______________

6. A policewoman caught the thief.

_______________

7. My mother will write a letter.

_______________

8. The child caught the ball.

_______________

9. His behavior irritates me.

_______________

10. The farmer ploughs the field .

_______________

**III. Change the following sentences into passive voice without using the agent 'By':**

1. She kept me waiting.

2. I expect good news.

3. Somebody has put the light on.

4. They sell computers here.

5. She has sold her car.

6. People will soon forget it.

7. We prohibit smoking.

8. They opened the restaurant only last week.

9. Suresh has defeated our team.

10. The police questioned him.

***Note:*** Sometimes verbs take both a direct and an indirect object in the active voice. When such verbs are changed to passive voice, the object may become the subject of the passive verb while the other is retained and is used as the object after a passive verb.

**Example**

i. *Active Voice:* Mr. Sinha teaches us physics.

*Passive Voice:* Physics is taught to us by Mr. Sinha.

or

We are taught Physics by Mr. Sinha.

ii. *Active Voice:* Who taught you child psychology?

*Passive Voice:* By whom was child psychology taught to you?

or

By whom were you taught child psychology?

**Now, change these sentences.**

iii. He handed her a chair.

iv. The conductor will give you a ticket.

____________________________________________

____________________________________________

____________________________________________

____________________________________________

Now, look at these sentences:

1. The door *is broken*.
2. She *is gone*. (= she *has gone*)

The verb *is broken* is in the passive voice.

But don't think that the verb *is gone* is in the passive voice. The verb 'go' is intransitive and only a transitive verb can be used in passive voice. For the same reason, the verbs in the following sentences are in the active voice.

She *is come.* She *is arrived.*

## Exercise

**Change the following sentences in active into sentences in the passive voice without using the agent 'by':**

1. They asked me my name.

2. They refused him admission.

3. I bought the child a sweet.

4. She found him guilty of murder.

5. You cannot pump the sea dry.

6. He saw the hurricane approaching.

7. He keeps me waiting.

8. They painted the house maroon.

9. She promised him a present.

10. I shall order the food.

**Now that you have understood how the active voice is changed into passive voice try changing the following sentences into active voice from the passive voice:**

1. She was praised by her teacher.

   ______________________________

2. The first inoculation was given by Dr. Edward Jenner.

   ______________________________

3. She was laughed at by all her friends.

   ______________________________

4. She was made the queen.

   ______________________________

5. Let the order be given.

   ______________________________

6. The city was destroyed by tornado.

   ______________________________

7. The prince was welcomed by the Prime Minister.

   ______________________________

8. The school was damaged by the riots.

   ______________________________

9. We shall be scolded by everyone.

   ______________________________

10. The work will be finished by Alexander in a fortnight.

    ______________________________

With this we come to the end of this section. Practise well and you will not find changing Voice tough.

## TENSE

Here we are at the most interesting section in verbs. It is called Tense. Tense comes from the Latin word TEMPUS, meaning 'time'. This tells us the time in which an action or condition has taken place and if this action has been completed or not.

Look at these sentences:

1. I *walk* in the garden.
2. I *walked* in the park with my friends.
3. I *shall walk* to college tomorrow.

In the first sentence, the verb *walk* refers to the **present** time.

In the second sentence, the verb *walked* refers to the time that is over i.e. time that is **past**.

In the third sentence, the verb *shall walk* refers to the time that is yet to take place. That is the time here refers to **future**.

Therefore a verb may refer to:

a. Present time

b. Past time

c. Future time



### Definitions

A verb that refers to the action in the present time is said to be in the **Present Tense.**

A verb that refers to the action that has happened in the past time is said to be in the **Past Tense.**

A verb that refers to the action that is supposed to happen in the future time is said to be in the **Future Tense.**

So, we realise there are three main Tenses.

The Past

The Present

The Future

# All About Verbs

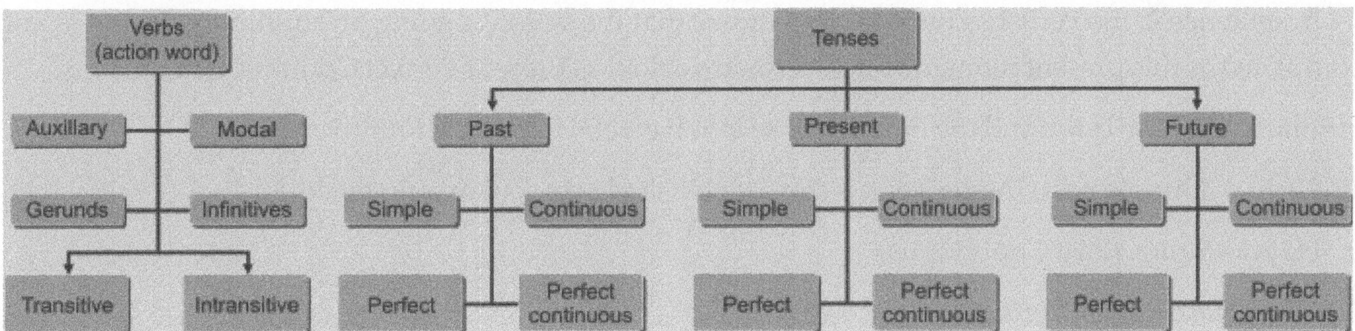


Some examples for all the three tenses:

Present Tense: Saurav *enjoys* playing.

Sophia *writes* neatly.

Past Tense: Saurav *enjoyed* playing.

Sophia *wrote* neatly.

Future Tense: Saurav *will enjoy* playing.

Sophia *will write* neatly.

Now look at these sentences:

1. He *takes* the book.
2. He *is taking* the book.
3. He *has taken* the book.
4. He *has been taking* the book.

The verbs in these sentences refer to the present time and thus are said to be in the present tense.

In sentence 1, the verb 'takes' shows that the action is mentioned simply and nothing is said about whether the action is completed or not. Therefore, verbs like these that are in the present and simple are called Simple Present Tense.

In sentence 2, the verb 'is taking' shows the action is not yet complete or it is still going on. That is it is continuous. Such verbs are called Present Continuous Tense.

In sentence 3, the verb 'has taken' shows that the action is finished, completed or perfect at the time of speaking. Such verbs are called as Present Perfect Tense.

In sentence 4, the verb 'has been taking' shows that the action is going on continuously and is not completed at this present moment. Such verbs are called as Present Perfect Continuous Tense.

Similarly the Past Tense and the Future Tense also have the following four forms.

1. He *took*. (Simple past) [**Note:** Took is the past tense of take. There is no taked.]
2. He was *taking*. (Past Continuous)
3. He *had taken*. (Past Perfect)
4. He *had been taking*. (Past Perfect Continuous)

**Future Tense**

1. He *shall take*. (Simple Future)
2. He *shall be taking*. (Future Continuous)
3. He *shall have taken*. (Future Perfect)
4. He *shall have been taking*. (Future Perfect Continuous)

Now, we understand that the Tense of a Verb shows not only the time of an action or event but also the state of an action referred to.



## Exercise

**Identify the verbs in the following sentences and name their tenses:**

1. The river flows under the bridge.
2. Nurse Varghese was making tea when the doctors arrived.
3. We have lived in Chennai for three years.
4. Santosh has been telephoning your friends since 6 o'clock.
5. She swam well.
6. When the group arrived at the station, the train had left.
7. They had been working very hard.
8. Ramya was walking to the post office.

9. I shall be eighteen this December.
10. Dr Shirin will be promoted by the end of the year.
11. Economists predict that the recession will have improved by next year.
12. By next July, I shall have been working here for two years.
13. Mohammed is a sailor.
14. It was snowing the whole day yesterday.
15. Sanjay has been in hospital for a week.
16. I went for a jog after I had finished the embroidery.
17. Sara went alone.
18. Nurse Sukanya was giving the injection to the baby.
19. Matron was getting angry at the carelessness of the patient's family.
20. The rains will stop in a day or two.



## USES OF TENSES

### Simple Present Tense

This is used in seven different situations.

1. To make clear a habit or a routine action like,

*Example:* Eric drinks hot water every morning.

I go to bed every night at 11:30.

The engine works smoothly.

2. To show general truths like,

*Example:* The sun rises in the east.

The nurse helps in the quick recovery of a patient.

There is no substitute for hard work.

3. In exclamatory sentences starting with here and there to show the action taking place in the present like,

*Example:* Here come the firefighters!

There blows the whale!

4. As a substitute for the Simple Past in a vivid narrative.

*Example:* The mother now rushes forward and picks up the baby.

Suddenly the consultant hurries to his chamber.

[This sort of talking is generally used in story-telling or while giving comments in sports or while narrating in the present the incidents that are taking place to another person. The other person may be in the same place or may be in a different place.]



5. It is used to indicate a future that is part of a plan or arrangement.

*Example:* I'll do the operation next week.

She leaves for Mysore by the next train.

We write the exam next Tuesday.

When does the hospital open?

6. It is used to introduce a quotation while writing an essay or letter or speed.

*Example:* Shakespeare says, "The world is a big stage and we are actors all."

7. It is used instead of the Simple Future Tense like,

*Example:* I shall wait till he finishes his lunch.

If it rains we shall take a taxi.

## Exercise

**Fill in the blank with a verb in the simple present form to complete each sentence:**

1. He ____________ five language.
2. Jayana is a nurse. She _______ Hindi.
3. Rejimo always _________ the door at night because it is warm.

4. This necklace __________ too much.

5. Everything in the nurses unit is very clean. One needs to ________ the rules of cleanliness there.

6. Mathew's job is boring because he ________ in the same room.

7. My mobile is not working. It ________ to be repaired soon.

8. They __________ to watch block buster movies.

9. Reshma _________ the orphanage every week.

10. They shall wait till you ______ your recording.

## Present Continuous Tense

This is used to show action taking place at the time of speaking. It also shows that the action is an on-going one, which means not yet completed.

*Example:* It is raining.

She is living in Mumbai.

This form of the present tense is used in the following ways:

1. To denote an action going on at the time of speaking.

*Example:* He is running (now is understood. Therefore it is not written).

The nurses are studying child psychology.

2. To show a temporary action that may not be actually happening at the time of speaking.

*Example:* I am reading 'Oliver Twist'. (But I am not reading it at this moment)

She is seeing David. (Meaning the lady in question is going steady/girlfriend of a man David).

Here seeing is not literally to be understood.

3. To show an action that is planned or arranged to take place in the near future.

*Example:* They are going to the movie in the evening.

His grand parents are arriving tonight.

She is going to dance tomorrow.

4. To show an obstinate habit. Like,

*Example:* My father is always chewing tobacco.

[This should not be confused with the simple present tense that shows habit. The present continuous tense that shows obstinate habit which persists in spite of advice or warning adverbs like always, continually, constantly are used.]

> ***Note:***
>
> Some verbs due to their meaning are not normally used in the continuous form. They are:
>
> i. verbs of perception: see, hear smell, notice, recognize.
>
> ii. verbs of appearing: appear, look, seem
>
> iii. verbs of emotion: want, wish, desire, feel, like, love, hate, hope, refuse, prefer
>
> iv. verbs of thinking: think, suppose, believe, agree, consider, trust, remember, forgot, know, understand, imagine, mean, mind.
>
> v. have (possess), own, possess, belong to, contain, consist of, be (except when used in the passive).



All these verbs are usually used in simple present tense. However, they may be used in the continuous tenses with a change of meaning.

*Example:* He is thinking of leaving the project. (This gives the meaning considering the idea of)

Nurse Sheeba is minding the baby while her sister is cooking. (This gives the meaning looking after)

## Exercise

**Fill in the blanks with present continuous tense. The verb is given in the bracket**

1. The bird ________________. (fly)
2. Nurse Ramon and Nurse Sheila ___________ in the ICU. (work)
3. Supradeep Pillai _____________ a journal. (read)
4 The tea is _____________, can you turn it off? (boil)
5. I'm _________ to bed now. Good night! (go)

**Write the following sentences in Simple Present Tense in Present Continuous Tense.**

1. I live with some friends.
2. He works hard.
3. I listen to radio.
4. John leaves his things all over the place.
5. Sharath stays at the Grand Pavilion.

**Now look at this sentence.**

- I always go to college by car.

Here 'always' shows a continuous habitual action. So the sentence is in Present Continuous Tense. Here one should not write or say

- I am always going to college by car.

Most non-English speakers make this mistake. The word 'going' does not give the same meaning as 'go'. Look at this sentence.

- I am going to Delhi. (Here going means 'leave; to another place, travel long distance)

Read NOTE given earlier on Verbs not usually used in continuous tense. When one has to use them the adverbs always, too often, more often than, constantly, continually are used.

- Savitha is always complaining.

This does not mean Savitha complains all the time. It means that she complains too often, more often than normal.

## Exercise

**Complete the sentences in present continuous tense by using 'always' where needed and the right form of verb given in the brackets:**

1. The bus ____________ on time. (leave)
2. Jenny is ____________ Robert. (see)
3. That bike is useless! It ___________ down. (break)
4. Shaina ____________ in Le Grande when she's in Sweden. (stay)
5. I'm ____________ something. (do)

## Present Perfect Tense

'Perfect' here means 'completed' or 'finished'. So Present Perfect Tense shows action that has been completed in the immediate past. But the time frame is still the present.

*Example:* John has gone to England.

Here the action of going is completed. But the time frame is 'now'.

The present perfect tense is used in four situations.

1. To show activities completed in the immediate past.

*Example:* She has just come in.

The bed has just been cleared.

2. To indicate past actions whose time is not specified or not definite.

*Example:* Have you read 'Oliver Twist'?

Ms. Suzi has been to Delhi.

3. To express past events whose effects are felt in the present than the action itself.

*Example:* Staff Nurse Rudi has finished his work. (Means now he is free)

The child has cut its finger. (Means the finger is bleeding now)

Notice the meaning shown in the bracket is understood. Therefore it is not written.

4. To show an action or event this has begun at sometime in the past and is continuing in the present moment.

*Example:* We have lived in Bengaluru for thirty-six years.

He has known him for a long time.

Rakesh hasn't seen Rahul for several years.

*Note:* Adverbs such as

1. Just, often, never, ever are used in Interrogative sentences or in questions in the Present Perfect Tense.
2. So far, till now, yet are used in negative as well as questions in the Present Perfect Tense.
3 Present Perfect is never used with adverbs of past time.

*Example:* She has gone to Jaisalmer yesterday.

## Exercises

**I. Fill in the blanks with present perfect tense with correct forms of verbs given in the bracket.**

1. She _________ her book. (lose)
2. They told me their names but I ___________ it. (forget)
3. I can't find my book, ________ you ________ it? (see)
4. The doctors ____________ the two patients with tuberculosis. (treat)
5. Shaista is on holiday. She's ___________ Dhanbad. (go)

**II. Read the situations and write sentences. Choose one of the verbs given below. The first sentence has been done as an example:**

sleep, clean, improve,

1. Nurse Rehand is looking for her watch. She can't find it. **She has lost her watch.**
2. The patient is sleeping now. He is sleeping for five hours now. ________________
3. Nurse Maria is cleaning the patient's wound. ____________________________
4. Tom's English wasn't very good. Now it is much better.______________________
5. Susan didn't have a pony tail last month. Now she has a pony tail. ___________________

We shall now go to the last topic in Present Tense.

## Present Perfect Continuous Tense

This is used to show an action which began at sometime in the past and is still continuing. There is a connection with *now.*

*Example:* They have been building the hospital for several months.

The children have been playing since 4 o' clock.

Sometimes this tense is used to show an action already finished. In such cases, the stress is on the continuity of the activity as an explanation of something.

This tense can be used to show actions repeated over a period of time. Like,

Steffanie is a very good gymnast. She's been doing it since she was six.

Every evening they meet in the same pub. They've been going there for years.

Let us notice the difference between Present Continuous Tense and Present Perfect Continuous Tense.

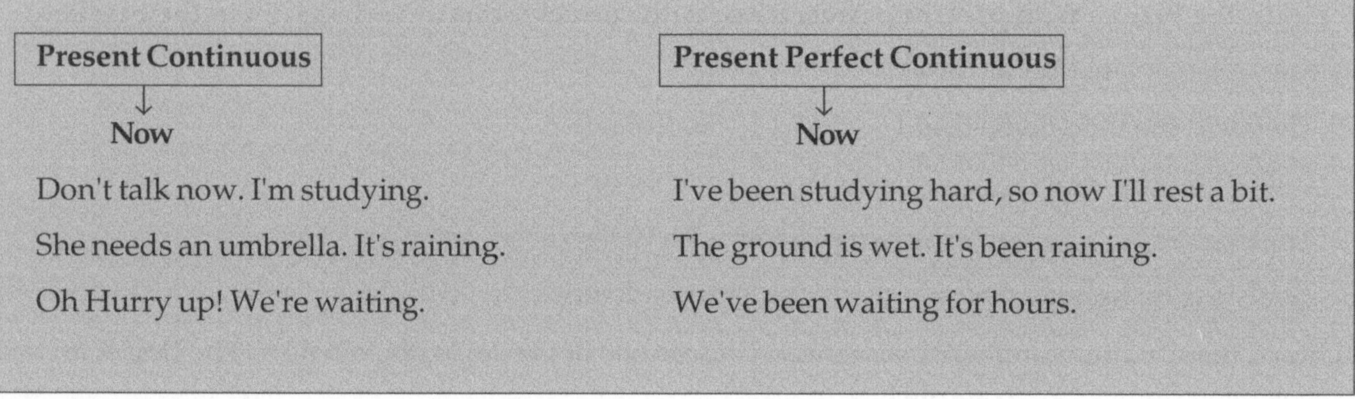

| **Present Continuous** | **Present Perfect Continuous** |
|---|---|
| ↓ **Now** | ↓ **Now** |
| Don't talk now. I'm studying. | I've been studying hard, so now I'll rest a bit. |
| She needs an umbrella. It's raining. | The ground is wet. It's been raining. |
| Oh Hurry up! We're waiting. | We've been waiting for hours. |



*Remember:* Present Perfect Continuous Tense:

| I / We / They / You / | Have | Been | Verb + ing |
|---|---|---|---|
| He / She / It | Has | | |
| Adding not after have/has gives negative sentence. | | | |
| They have not been sleeping. She has not been sleeping. | | | |

This tense form cannot be used in passive form.

*Example:* "Why are your fingers so messy?" - 'I have been finger-painting'

In other words in this tense form emphasis is on the Christmas card.

*Exercise:* Length of time a certain action has gone on continuously.

## Exercise

**I. Complete the given sentences with present perfect continuous tense. Verbs are given in the bracket:**

1. It __________ (Rain).
2. He's out of breaths. ___________ he ___________? (run)
3. Lizzie is very tired. She's _____________ very hard. (work)
4. I ____________ to Matron about the problem and she thinks that it can be solved. (talk)
5. How long _________ you __________ nursing? (learn)

**II. Write a question for each situation, the first one has been done for you.**

1. Josh looks thirsty. You ask: (you/work in the Sun?)
   Have you been working in the sun?
2. You have just arrived to meet a friend who is waiting for you. You ask (you/wait/long?)

______________________________________________________________________

3 Mother meets son coming through the gate. His face and hands are dirty. She asks: (what/you/do?)

______________________________________________________________________

4. A patient has come into the clinic with a bleeding wound.
   You ask: (how long/wound/bleed/happened?)

______________________________________________________________________

5. A neighbour is now living in a different locality. You want to know 'How long ....?'
   You ask: (how long/you live/in ________?)

______________________________________________________________________

With this we have come to know about Present Tense. We shall now know about the different forms of Past Tense.

## Simple Past Tense

Simple Past Tense is used to show an action that is completed in the past time. Like,

I received the parcel a month ago.

You can see that the action has taken place 30 days ago. The time indicated in Simple Past Tense may be in the distant or immediate past.

*Example:* Nurse Abheesh *sold* his bike yesterday.

I *left* the office fifteen minutes ago.

Chandra Gupta Maurya *ruled* India more than 2500 years ago.

He *left* college last year.

This tense is used to show past habits.

*Example:* He *worked* for eight hours every day.

She always *carried* a hand bag.

When this tense is used without an adverb of time, then time may be either implied or indicated by the situation.

*Example:* I *learnt* Marathi in Pune.

She *didn't* sleep well. (i.e. last night)



## Exercise

**Fill in the blanks with simple past tense form of the verb given in the bracket:**

1. I ____________ English yesterday. (study)
2. Wolfgang Amadeus Mozart ________ an Austrian musician and composer. (is)
3. Mozart ________ composing at the age of five. (start)
4. She works in a hospital now. Before that she ____________ in a shop. (work)
5. We _______ nurses Abhilesh and Joan in a concert a few days ago. (see)
6. It was cold, so Revathi _________ the window. (shut)

*7. They _________Jennifer to the party, so she _______ ______. (did, invite, did, go)

*8. I ____________ anything. (did, do)

9. Professor Sarathy __________ angry because students ________ late. (is, is)
10. 'How did you learn to drive?' The driver _________ me. (teach)

**(negative sentences 7 & 8)*

**Remember: Simple Past Tense:**

| | | Example Word |
|---|---|---|
| Positive | I, we, You, He, She, It, They | Took |
| Question | Did I, We, You, He, She, It, They | take? |
| Negative | I, We, You, He, She, It, They | did not take (didn't take) |
| Passive Voice | I, He, She, It | was taken |
| | We, You, They | were taken |

## Past Continuous Tense

This is used to–

1. Denote an action, event or state going on at some time in the past. The time of action may or may not be indicated.

*Example:*

We *were listening* to the music all evening.

(Usually Asian Students say 'whole evening' or 'entire evening'. This is wrong usage. All evening is correct.)

Let us know the sentence better.

Since 'we' is plural the 'be' form verb in the plural is - were.

Listen is the root verb or main verb. Adding 'ing' shows that the action is continuous. But it is so in the past time. Thus the verb 'were listening' is in past continuous tense.

You might have recognized that the present continuous tense also has 'ing' added to the verb. This may make you say continuous action is denoted by adding 'ing' (verb + ing). Yes it is true. But one must take enough care with the 'be' form verb before the continuous verb. If is, was, were, get mixed up, then the sentence goes for a toss.

Let us continue with the examples.

It was *getting* darker.

The child was *crying* in the ICU all night.

When I saw Dr. Able, he *was playing* chess.

2. With 'always', 'continually', etc. to show persistent habits in the past.

*Example:* Grand mother *was always grumbling* about the house.

Her brother *was always smoking* cigarettes.

3. Past continuous is used with the simple past tense to define one action in relation to another in the past. Here the actual time of action may or may not be indicated.

*Example:* Dr. Suresh *was instructing* the patient about his diet when I *walked* in.

Here *was instructing* is in past continuous tense. *Walked* is in simple past tense.

You will notice that the action of walking inside was completed but the instructing was in progress.

Now look at these sentences.

a. They *were walking* when they met Mr. Shastry.

b. They *walked* when they met Mr. Shastry.



They will notice that in sentence 'a' the walking was in progress when they met Mr. Shastry, while in sentence 'b' the walking began and ended when they met Mr. Shastry. That is, only when they saw Mr. Shastry, they walked up to him. So, the action of walking began & ended with the sighting of Mr. Shastry.

4. Past continuous tense is used all by itself (without the presence of past simple tense) to show that an action was going on for a specific/certain period of time in the past.

*Example:* He *was heating* the iron for three hours.

Matron O'Reily *was packing* her things the whole day. She *was shifting* to a new house.

5. Sometimes to show two or more past actions/activities were happening at the same time, two or more verbs, all in the past continuous tense is used.

*Example:*

i. The students *were writing* the exam while the invigilator *was going* around the room.

ii. While father *was watering* the plants, I *was washing* the dog.

iii. The 'last Retreat' was playing; the six foot soldiers on either side of the border *were marching* towards each other and as the assembled crowd was watching, the soldiers closed the gates at the border-crossing.

## Exercise

**Fill up the blanks with past continuous tense form of the verbs given in the brackets:**

1. Yesterday Sue and Jime __________ tennis. (play)
2. This time last year I _____________ in Upper Manali. (trek)
3. Sister Rashida ___________ when the phone rang. (watch)
4. Dr. Raghavendra burnt his hand while he _______ the dinner. (cook)
5. Sabina fell asleep while she __________ for her friend. (wait)
6. Tenzing and Hillary _________ (plan) the assault to the peak while they ________ (take) shelter from the snowstorm in their tent.
7. While Nurse Dhanooja __________the syringe (sterilize), nurse Reenamol _________ on the intercom. (talk)
8. Student Nurse Mayoori ______________ excited to participate in her first surgical duty. (feel)
9. I _______ on a brown frisky horse on the steep slopes of the Shiwalik ranges last summer. (ride)
10. Banisha _________ child care (study) while Mathew ___________ about postnatal care. (read)



## Past Perfect Tense

1. This tense shows an action completed before a certain moment in the past.

*Example:* I met Dr. Muttanna in Bangalore in 1976. I had seen her last five years before.

Words like **before, after, when, as soon as, by the time, until** show the relationship in time between the actions completed before a certain moment in the past.

*By the time* the students arrived the college was painted.

The exams were over on May 31st. The students left for home after a week.

2. When two actions have happened in the past, it may be necessary to show which of the two actions happened first. Past perfect tense is used in such cases. The simple past is used in one clause and the past perfect in the other.

*Example:* When I *reached* the station the train *had left.*

Simple Past — Past Perfect

Rahul *had done* his homework when Shweta *came* to see him.

Past Perfect                Simple Past

At this point, you may be confused between present perfect tense and past perfect tense. Let us clarify any confusions lingering in your mind.

In a way, we can say that this tense talks of past in the past. It is used to refer to action at a time before a point of time that is already in the past.

Look at the two sentences below:

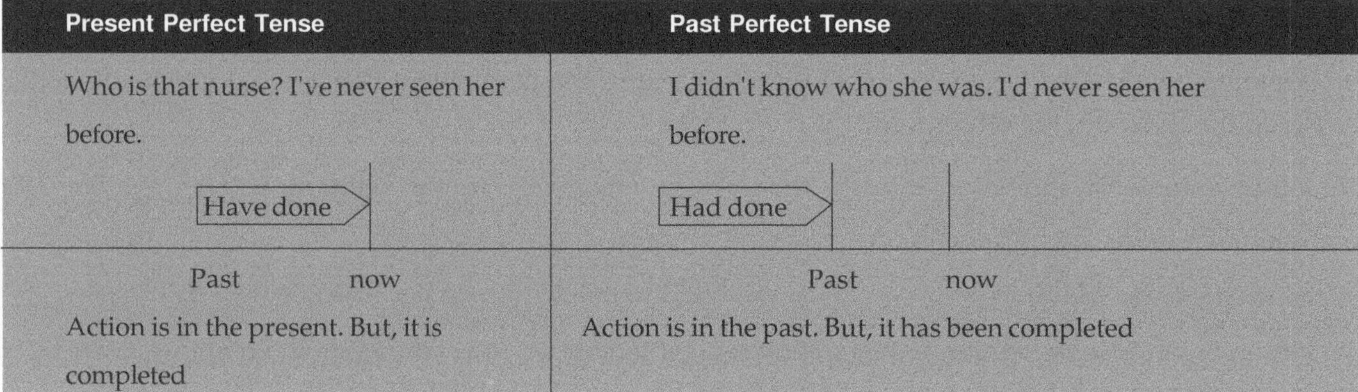

| Present Perfect Tense | Past Perfect Tense |
|---|---|
| Who is that nurse? I've never seen her before. | I didn't know who she was. I'd never seen her before. |
| Have done | Had done |
| Past now | Past now |
| Action is in the present. But, it is completed | Action is in the past. But, it has been completed |



The purpose of this tense is to put events or actions in a chronological order and to make it clear which action took place first.

**Look at these two sentences:**

1. When we *arrived* at the canteen, the cook left.
2. When we *arrived* at the canteen, the cook had left.

In the first sentence our arrival at the station coincided with the cook leaving (here left is to be taken as leaving for the day after the job was done. The meaning here is not leaving the job to take on a new job). We could have talked to the cook (in terms of exchanging pleasantries) or we could have missed seeing the cook. Notice that both the finite verbs are in the past simple tense.

In the second sentence it is clear that we missed seeing the cook. Cook left first and then, minutes later, we arrived at the canteen.

**Remember:**

| | | Past Perfect Form |
|---|---|---|
| Positive | I/We/You/He/She/It/They | had taken |
| Negative | I/We/You/He/She/It/They | had not (hadn't) taken |
| Question | Had I/We/You/He/She/It/They | taken? |
| Passive Voice | I/We/You/He/She/It/They | had been taken |

## Exercises

**I. Fill in the blanks with past perfect tense form of the verbs given in the brackets:**

1. When nurse Lohith arrived at the party, Samantha ________ already ________ home. (go)
2. When she got home yesterday, she found that somebody ______________ into the house. (break)
3. The doctor ______ just _______ home when I phoned. (reach)
4. The store-room was dirty. They ___________ ___________ it for weeks. (clean)
5. At first he thought he ____ ________ the right thing, but he soon realized that he ____ _________ a serious mistake. (do), (make)
6. By the time his relatives arrived at the hospital, Mr. Suri ______ ________ ________ into the operation theatre. (be + take)
7. They _____ _______ that certain details were missed in the analysis. (-ve + send)
8. Staff Nurse Tandin __________ ___________ a woolen blanket at the foot of the bed. (place)
9. Rajeshwari _________ already _________ the contraceptive pill before I could warn her of its side effects. (take)
10. As soon as the surgeon ________ __________ his gloves he ________ his hands thoroughly under running water. (remove), (wash)

**II. Use the sentences on the left to complete the paragraphs on the right. These sentences are in the order in which they happened- 1 then 2 then 3 but your paragraph begins with the underlined sentence. This is where you need past perfect tense.**

| | |
|---|---|
| (i) 1. Somebody broke into the shop during the night. | We arrived at work in the morning and |
| 2. We arrived at work in the morning. | found somebody____________________ |
| 3. We called the police | in the office during the night.So we |
| . | __________________________________. |
| (ii) 1. Sara went out | Tom tried to phone Sara this morning |
| 2. Tom tried to phone her this morning | but ____________________no answer. She |
| 3. There was no answer. | ______________________out. |
| (iii) 1. Jasmine came back from EBC trek a week ago. | I met Jasmine a few days ago. She ______ ______________________just ____________ |
| 2. I met her the same day. | she ___________________________________. |
| 3. She looked well. | |

(iv)

(v)

Let us now go to the last part of past tense form.

## Past Perfect Continuous Tense

This tense is similar to the past perfect tense. This too denotes actions in past time at a moment in the past. But, unlike the past perfect tense, the continuous tense stresses the duration of the action in the past. Due to this, this tense usually goes with a time expression starting with 'since' or 'for'.

**Note:** There is no passive form of this tense.

In other words, the past perfect continuous tense is used for an action that started before a particular time in the past and continued up to that time.

*Example:* At that time she *had been writing* a novel for two years.

When Mr. Radhakishen came to the nursing college in 1975, Mrs. Anna Phadnis *had* already *been teaching* there for five years.

Ms Subbalakshmi the famous Carnatic Vocalist was a prodigy. She *had been singing* since her sixth year.

When the boys came into the house, their clothes were dirty, their hair were untidy and one of them had a black eye. They'd *been fighting.*

**Look at this sentence**

Our game of chess was interrupted. *We'd been* playing for about half an hour when guests came home.

You can say that something *had been happening* for a period of time before something else happened.

From all these examples you can say **had been -ing** shows the past perfect continuous tense form.

**Let us compare present perfect continuous and past perfect continuous.**

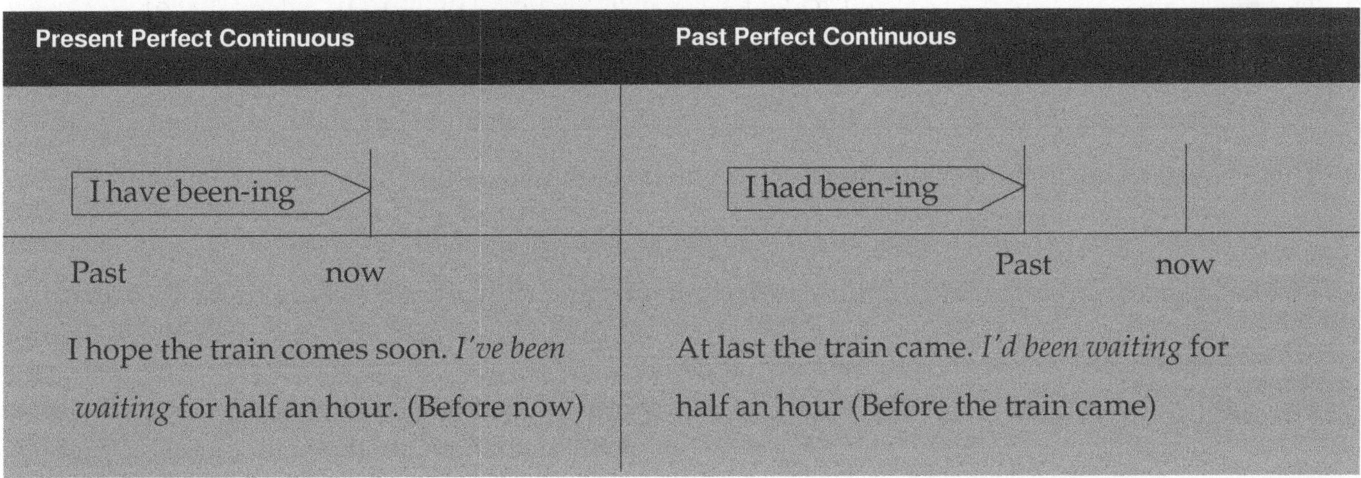

| Present Perfect Continuous | Past Perfect Continuous |
|---|---|
| I have been-ing | I had been-ing |
| Past now | Past now |
| I hope the train comes soon. *I've been waiting* for half an hour. (Before now) | At last the train came. *I'd been waiting* for half an hour (Before the train came) |

You can form a sentence that has both past continuous tense and the past perfect continuous tense.

*Example:*

It *wasn't raining* when they come home. The sun *was shining*. But it *had been raining,* so the ground was wet.

**Remember:**

| | | |
|---|---|---|
| Positive: | I/We/You/He/She/It/they | had been talking |
| Negative: | I/We/You/He/She/It/they | had not (hadn't) been talking. |
| Question: | Had I/We/You/He/She/It/they | been talking? |

## Exercises



**I. Read the situations and make sentences from the words in brackets. One has been done to show you. Use only the past perfect continuous tense form.**

1. She was very tired when she arrived home. (she/work/hard all day)

   **She had been working hard all day.**

2. The two men come into the hospital. They had rackets and they were both very tired. (they/play/ tennis)

   ______________________________

3. There was nobody in the hall but there was a smell of tobacco. (somebody/smoke/in the hall)

   ______________________________

4. I woke up in the middle of the night. I was frightened and didn't know where I was. (I/dream)

   ______________________________

5. The climbers were tired when they reached base camp. (they/skiing/down slope)

   ______________________________

**II. Fill up the blanks with the correct form of past perfect continuous tense. Verbs are given in brackets:**

1. ______ I been ______ (write) to him? Who said that?
2. We _______ _______ ______ ______ (swim) in the river.

3. They ______ _______ ________ their college last evening. (describe)
4. Jelaja _____ ______ ______ of a rosy life for herself. (dream)
5. It ______ ______ ______ function to honor the Mt. Everest summiteers. (glitter)
6. She _____ _____ _____ for the address for an hour. (look)
7. If you ____ not _____ _______ for the bus in the Clark bus stand. You would not have been ruffed. (wait)
8. Senior Nurse Jagin ____ _____ ______ for eighteen years when she thought of changing her profession. (work)
9. All the doctors in the city ____ _____ _____ late hours last year when the news of swine flu hit the headlines. (work)
10. Simon ____ ___ _______ with his pet before he jumped into the lake to save the small boy. (play)

With this you have come to the end of past tense form of verbs. Your next unit is on the use of different forms of future tense.



## FUTURE TENSE

As the term suggests, this tense shows possible actions in the future. There are two kinds/forms of future. Yes, you read it right. There are two kinds/forms of future. One is pure or colourless future. The other is coloured future. Both these are found in simple future tense. Let us know more about this tense.

### Simple Future Tense

This is used for an action that is yet (has still) to take place:

*Example:* She shall see me tomorrow.

Tomorrow is Tuesday.

Now in these actions which have not yet taken place, we have pure or colourless future. This is an action or event that happens because it has to happen or in other words it cannot help happening. There is no way a human being can control the action or event from taking place.

*Example:* Nurse Simon's birthday is on 18th may. He *shall* be 26.

The day-after-tomorrow *will* be a busy day.

Dawn *will* break soon.

The rains *will fill* the rivers to capacity.

The operation *will be* performed tomorrow.

Now pure futures like those you read above are few to experience. They have least to do with people or individuals. Most are the kind of future actions/events that are made to depend on external factors.

*Example:*

Mother *shall let* you go out to play if you have finished your homework.

They *will get* the electronics goods when they go to Singapore.

A coloured future is an action or event that takes place because someone wants/wishes/intends it to happen. Like,

I *will go* on a boating trip next week. (Because I want to go)

You *will hold* this for me until I pay the bill. (It is my order for you)

They *shall not* go to the party. (I shall see to it they'll not go)

(shan't)

'Shall' and 'will' denote both kinds of future.

## Exercise

**Fill in the blanks with 'will' or 'shall'. The sentences may be in pure or coloured future.**

1. It _______ rain tomorrow.
2. Tomorrow ______ be a challenging day.
3. They ______ not go unpunished.
4. Do you think it ______ be sunny tomorrow?
5. The nurse _____ work on all days if they are paid overtime to give up their holidays. (this is just a practice sentence & not to be taken seriously)

6. How late in the night _____ the shops open?
7. They ____ not go to the movie tomorrow.
8. I ____ not go to see the movie tomorrow.
9. You _____ have your book back tomorrow.
10. "Ask anything you want and you _____ have it," says the king.

## Future Continuous Tense

This tense has no passive form. This is more of pure future forms. This tense denotes an action as 'going on' at some time in the future time.

*Example:* When I get to the office, my work *will be lying* on my table.

I *shall be playing* chess then.

This is also used to show a future event or experience happening as a natural course without intentions and planning interrupting it.

*Example:*

Mr. Prakash *will be going* on leave for the summer months as his children *will be waiting* to visit their grandparents during their summer vacations.

Smt. Radha Kashyap *will be retiring* by the end of the year.

This is also used to denote distant future. Like,

I wonder what she *will be doing* two years from now.

This tense can also show future to be very close to the present. Like,

The plastering done and soon the painters *will be painting* the house.

## Exercise

**Fill in the blanks with future continuous tense form of the verbs given in the brackets:**

1. I _________ (be + stay) here till Monday.
2. She ________ us next month. (be + meet)

3. You _________ from the recruiter soon. (be + hear)

4. _____ she ________ her laptop today? (be + use)

5. It _______ all the instructions to the last letter. (be + follow)

## Future Perfect Tense

This tense is used to indicate the completion of an action by a certain time in the future.

*Example:* She *shall have written* the book by that time.

Before you go to talk to him, he *will have left* the place.

This tense is usually used to make predictions. Like,

According to the traders, the gold price in the country *will have risen* by a further 1% by the end of this year.

Scientist say that by the end of two years global warming *will have melted* 1.5% of the polar ice cap

This tense form has passive form.

**Remember:**

| Form | | Verb |
|---|---|---|
| Question | Will I/We/You/She/he/It/They | have spoken? |
| Negative | I/We/You/She/he/It/They | will not have spoken |
| Positive | I/We/You/She/He/It/They | will have spoken |
| Passive Voice | I/We/You/She/He/It/They | will not (won't) have been taken |

## Exercise

**Fill in the blanks with future perfect tense form of the verbs given in the brackets:**

1. If she saves $ 10 a day, in a year's time she _______ (save) $ 3650.
2. Studies have shown that child obesity _______ (rise) by 5% in 2 years.
3. According to entomologists 2% of insects __________ (extinct) by 2080 AD.

4. His Ph.D _________ (complete) by that time.
5. By the end of next year you __________(finish) the nursing course.

## Future Perfect Continuous Tense

This tense denotes an action as being in progress over a period of time that will end in the future.

*Example:*

By next August we *shall have been living* here for eight years.

When Simone gets her degree, she *will have been studying* at RJB University for four years.

We must remember that future perfect tense and future perfect continuous tense are not used as much as the simple future. But, they are used in certain situations as you have studied.

Present simple tense and present continuous are also used to show the future time frame. 'Will' and 'shall' are used to show future tense.

As we do not often use the future perfect continuous tense, exercise has been omitted.

With this we come to the end of tenses. Wish you luck in learning and using the different time frames in your life. Remember to practise as much as possible one read does not make you expert in the usage.



## INFINITIVE

Observe the sentences:

1. They always *find* fault with me.
2. They always try to *find* fault with me.

Let us take sentence 1. *They* always *find* fault with me.

Here the verb has *'they'* for subject. So, the verb is limited by person and number. Such a verb is called a **Finite verb.**

Let us take sentence 2. They always *try to find* fault with me.

An Infinitive is a non-finite verb. This is because it by itself cannot make a statement about a subject.

*Example:* She *to go* college.

They *to go* swimming.

It is proper to say the same thing as:

She has *to go* to college.

They have *to go* swimming.

The first set of sentences does not make statements because they are not proper sentences. The second sets are proper sentences and they make statements. This is because the first sets have a non-finite verb *'to go'*. The second sets have a finite verb each.

**Note #1:** A finite verb expresses person and number and has more than one form.



*Example:* She is *coming* home. (3rd person, singular)

I am *coming* home. (1st person, singular)

They *are coming* home. (3rd person, plural)

A non- finite verb has only one form. Let us see the non-finite verb 'to hear'.

*Example:* She is coming *to hear* the music.

I am coming *to hear* the music.

They are coming *to hear* the music.

**Note #2:** Only finite verbs can be put in various tenses.

**Note #3:** The infinitive consists of the simple form of the verb usually but not always preceded by the sign *'to'*.

*Example:* He is keen to *eat all* the sweets.

An infinitive phrase is a word-group with no subject-predicate and headed by an infinitive. This may function as a noun, as an adjective or as an adverb.

*Example*: *To forget a name* when in company can be very embarrassing.

For once she decided *to deal money*.

After certain verbs like *bid, let, make, need, dare, see, hear,* we use the infinitive without *to.*

*Example:* *Bid* her *go* there.

*Let* her *sit* here.

*Make* him *run.*

They *need* not *come* today.

You *dare* not *do it.*

I *saw* you *doing* it.

I *hear* her *cry.*

**Note #4:** The infinitive without *to* is also used after the verbs *shall, will, do, did, should, would, may, might.*



## Exercises

**I. Fill in the blanks using the correct form of infinitive. The verbs are given in the brackets.**

1. Can you _______ the stars? (count)
2. I _______ see you. (be + come)
3. She is sorry _______ this. (hear)
4. Full many a flower is born _______ unseen. (blush)
5. Everybody wishes _______life. (enjoy)
6. _______ the truth, I quite forgot my promise. (tell)
7. We eat _______. (live)
8. Apples are good _______. (eat)
9. The girls are eager _______. (learn)
10. This is not the time _______. (play)
11. This apartment is _______. (let)
12. _______ is human. (error)

13. I like _______ hockey. (play)
14. The chief guest is about _______. (speak)
15. _______ our parents is our duty. (respect)

**II. Combine the parts given under I and II below to form meaningful acceptable sentences:**

| I | II |
|---|---|
| She has a large family | to go abroad. |
| He expressed a wish | to feel ashamed. |
| I have no plans | to check the price-rise. |
| There is no reason | to tackle the difficulty. |
| Give them some books | to support. |
| They know the way | to see his mother. |
| The government took steps | to read in their spare time. |



1. ______________________________________________.
2. ______________________________________________
3. ______________________________________________
4. ______________________________________________
5. ______________________________________________
6. ______________________________________________
7. ______________________________________________

**III. Form at least ten correct and meaningful sentences with the help of the table given below:**

| Subject | Verb | To - infinitive showing purpose |
|---|---|---|
| He | got up | to meet his friend |
| They | ran | to welcome the visitor |
| Abheesh | came | to visit the mall |
| The professor | went | to get the news |

1. ____________________

2. ____________________

3. ____________________

4. ____________________

5. ____________________

6. ____________________

7. ____________________

8. ____________________

9. ____________________

10. ____________________

We now move on to the Participle.

## PARTICIPLE

Observe this sentence:

*Hearing* the sound, the girl woke up.

The word *hearing* describes the noun girl as an adjective does. But this word '*hearing*' is formed from the verb hear. Therefore, the word hearing takes the nature of both a verb and an adjective, and is called a **participle**.

**Definition:** A participle is that form of the verb which takes the nature of both, a verb and an adjective.

or

A participle is a word which is partly a verb and partly an adjective.

At this point do not get confused with a Gerund. A gerund and a participle are two different forms though they end with -ing. Read on and all your confusions will be clarified.

**Look at these sentences:**

1. They met a boy *carrying* a basket of chickens.
2. Loudly *knocking* on the door, he ordered the people to come out.

The above sentences represent an action as going on or incomplete. The verbs ending in -ing are in the present. So they are called present participles.

Observe the sentences given below:

*Blinded* by rain, they fell into disorder.

Time *misspent* is time lost.

*Driven* by hunger, the child stole the bread.

These sentences show completed action or state of the thing spoken of. Such verbs are called past participles. You will notice that the past participle usually ends in -ed,-t,-en or -n. [At the end of verbs you have a list of past participles given in this chapter.]

Besides the present and past participle, there is another participle. It is called the perfect participle. This represents an action as completed at some past time.

*Example: Having rested*, they continued their journey.

*Having rested* tells that the group of people travelling together stopped their travel for sometime, relaxed and then continued on their journey. The action 'rest' is completed in the past time. Therefore, it is perfect participle.

As this is beyond your syllabus we shall not go into details.

Present participle and past participle is all that you need to know at this stage.

## Errors in the Use of Participles

As participle is a verb-adjective, it must be attached to some noun or pronoun. That is, it should have a subject.

The following sentences are incorrect.

1 *Being* a hot day, I remained in the house.

2. *Sitting* on the wall, a snake bit him.

3. *Entering* the studio, the light was dazzling.

Notice that in sentence 2, it reads as if the snake was sitting on the wall. The same way sentence 3 gives the impression that a dazzling light entered the studio. We should therefore re-write the sentences as shown:

1. It being a hot day, I remained in the house.
2. While he was *sitting* on the wall, the snake bit him.
3. When I *entered* the studio, the light was dazzling

   OR

*Entering* the studio, I found the light dazzling.

## Exercises

**I. Pick out the participle in each of the following sentences and identify the participle(present or past participle):**

1. She saw the hurricane approaching.
2. Hearing a cough in the silent corridor, I became alert.
3. Considering the facts, Bhopal gas tragedy victims received scant justice.
4. Being dissatisfied, the customers stopped going to that shop.
5. The rain came pouring down in torrents.
6. The thief fled from the scene hearing the voices of people.
7. The fat of the body is fuel laid away for use.
8. Books read in childhood seem like old friends.
9. Seeing the sunshine, I ran out of the house.
10. It began to snow as we set foot in Namche Bazaar.

**II. Combine the following pairs of sentences by making use of participle:**

One has been done as an example.

**The fairy took pity on the poor girl. She turned her into a princess.**

**Taking pity on the poor girl, the fairy turned her into a princess.**

1. The watchman opened the gate. They entered.

_______________

2. She started early. She arrived at noon.

_______________

3. We met a doctor. He was carrying huge books.

_______________

4. A passenger alighted from the Mumbai Train. She fell over a bag on the platform.

_______________

5. Maria met her sister on the street. She asked her where she was going.

_______________

6. The patient staggered back. He sank to the ground.

_______________

7. The prescription was badly written. I had great difficulty in making out its contents.

_______________

8. A hungry fox saw some bunches of grapes. They were hanging from a vine.

_______________

9. The plane was delayed by volcanic ash. It landed in the airport a week later.

_______________

10. The chicken coop was open. The chickens were stolen.

_______________

## GERUNDS

Look at this sentence.

*Singing* is her favourite hobby.

The word *singing* is formed from the verb sing, by adding -ing. Another aspect to notice here is that 'singing' is used as the subject of a verb and thus does the work of a noun. (Remember that every sentence has a subject, object/predicate, where the subject is always a noun.) It is therefore a Verb-Noun. Such a word is called as a Gerund.

To understand this, let us observe some more sentences.

1. *Reading* epics is a favourite pastime in this house.
2. Nurse Medha likes *reading* novels.
3. They are fond of *eating* pizzas.

Let us take sentence 1. Here *'reading'* is the Gerund. Here the gerund is like a noun—it is the subject of a verb. Along with this, like a verb, it also takes an object. Therefore, it shows that it also has the force of the verb (action word).

Let us take sentence 2. Here *'reading'* is the Gerund. It is placed just before the sentence ends. Thus, it is the object of a verb. Yet, it does have the characteristic of a verb.

Let us take sentence 3. Here *'eating'* is the Gerund. It is working like a noun and is governed by a preposition. But like a verb, it also takes an object.

After these explanations, we can define a gerund now.

**Definition:** A Gerund is that form of the verb which ends in -ing, and has the force of a Noun and a Verb.

> *Note #1:* Both the gerund and the infinitive have the verb-noun form and thus have the same use. Therefore, in many sentences either of them may be used without any special difference in meaning.

*Example:* Teach me *to sing.*

Teach me *singing.*

To see is *to believe*.

Seeing is *believing*.

***Note #2:*** Both the gerund and the present participle end in -ing. One must be careful in using them. Gerund is a verb-noun. Present participle is a verb-adjective.

*Examples:*

| **Gerund** | **Present participle** |
|---|---|
| 1. He is fond of *playing* hockey. | 1. *Playing* hockey, he gained friends. |
| 2. The young lady was tired of *running*. | 2. *Running* along the road, she noticed a snake slithering away. |
| 3. Seeing is *believing*. | 3. *Seeing*, she believed. |



***Note #3:*** In compound nouns like walking-stick, frying-pan, writing-table; walking, frying, writing are gerunds.

## Use of the Gerund

A gerund being a verb-noun may be used in the following ways:

1. As subject of a verb.

   *Example: Reading* epics is a favourite pastime in this house.

2. Object of a preposition.

   *Examples:* She is tired of *waiting*.

   They are fond of *writing*.

   He has an aversion to *trekking*.

   We were prevented from *meeting* the principal.

3. Complement of a verb.

   *Example: Seeing* is *believing*.

## Exercises

**I. Point out the participles and gerunds in the following sentences:**

1. The boys were found fighting desperately for the first bench.
2. She has ruined her sight by reading in dim light.
3. They met a magician standing on his head.
4. Asking questions is easier than answering them.
5. Waving their hands and flags, the people cheered the cricket team.
6. Singing in the corridor is banned.
7. Jumping over the low wall, the dog escaped.
8. The cheat spends his time in cheating people.
9. I will not regret choosing to be a nurse.
10. Nursing is a noble profession.

**II. Fill in the blanks with gerunds of the verb given in the brackets:**

1. He could give up ____________. (smoke)
2. They enjoy ____________ (watch) films.
3. It was no use ____________ (call) the police.
4. Stop ____________ (talk). Don't you see I am learning to sing?
5. He failed to report for work and was punished for ____________ (remain) absent without notice.
6. He said he didn't mind ____________ (spend) a little extra money.
7. I always dreamt of ____________ (drive) an ambulance.
8. Teachers and parents never stop ____________ (advise) us about academic achievements.
9. My family is ____________ (wait) to see my sister who is in USA.
10. The nurse is ____________ (inject) the medicine as per the doctor's instructions.

Here we come to the end of gerunds. The next topic is strong and weak verbs, regular and irregular verbs.

## STRONG AND WEAK VERBS, REGULAR AND IRREGULAR VERBS

Earlier we came across kinds of verbs (transitive and intransitive). Now we shall know the parts of the verbs. The principal parts of a verb in English are:

The Present Tense

The Past Tense, and

The Past Participle.

Notice these:

| Present tense | Past tense |
|---|---|
| walk | walked |
| laugh | laughed |
| want | wanted |
| believe | believed |
| spend | spent |

These verbs form their past tense by adding -ed or -d or -t to the present. Such verbs are called weak verbs.

Observe these now:

| Present tense | Past tense |
|---|---|
| come | came |
| see | saw |
| write | wrote |
| begin | began |
| speak | spoke |
| know | knew |

These verbs form their past tense by changing the inside without adding -ed,-d or -t to the present tense. Such verbs which form past tense without having anything added are called strong verbs.

Now look at these verbs.

| Present tense | Past tense |
|---|---|
| sell | sold |
| bring | brought |
| buy | bought |
| catch | caught |
| seek | sought |
| teach | taught |

These verbs need the addition of -d or -t even though the inside vowel is changed to form the past tense. Such verbs are termed as weak verbs. Thus, we have the definition:

***Definition #1:*** Verbs that form their past tense by merely changing the vowel in the body of the present tense without adding and ending are called **Strong verbs**.

***Definition #2:*** Verbs that form their past tense by adding -ed,-d or -t to the present tense, with or without any inside vowel-change are called **Weak verbs.**

These two terms 'Strong verbs' and 'Weak verbs' roughly correspond to 'Regular verbs' and 'Irregular verbs'. To know the thin line that divides these terms is interesting but beyond the scope of this book.

After having read this, you will ask what are 'Regular and Irregular verbs'?

Here is your answer.

**Regular verbs:** These are verbs that form their past tense by adding -d,-t,-ed bound without any other change.

| Like- | Present tense | Past tense |
|---|---|---|
| | walk | walked |
| | state | stated |

**Irregular verbs:** These are verbs that form their past tense irregularly by a vowel change. These are verbs which have the same form in both the tenses.

| Like- | Present tense | Past tense |
|---|---|---|
| | tell | told |
| | sing | sang |
| | put | put |
| | cut | cut |

**[There is no putted or cutted in the English language]**

A list of present tense, past tense and past participle form is given here. It has both strong and weak, regular and irregular verbs.

Once again, I stress that to know the thin line that divides these terms is interesting but beyond the scope of this book.



## Exercises

**I. In the following sentences, change the verb to the past tense:**

1. Dr. Bhat writes to his parents every week.

______________________________

2. The widow slams shut.

______________________________

3. She sings melodiously.

______________________________

4. The patients sit in the waiting room.

______________________________

5. Their voice shakes with emotion.

______________________________

6. I do it on my own free will.

______________________________

7. Nurse Rudy asks the mother to stop crying.

______________________________

8. The doctors are tired working for 48 hours without rest.

_______________________________________________

9. The television news clips of the air crash site brought gasps of horror from viewers.

_______________________________________________

10. This poem takes too much time to finish.

_______________________________________________

**II. Fill in the blanks with past tense or past participle forms of verbs given:**

1. It is years since I _______her. She has _______ her best days. (see)
2. Of late, the custom has _______ into disuse. (fall)
3. The lot _______ upon them. (fall)
4. At the wedding reception the toast was _______ with great enthusiasm. (drink)
5. Hindi is _______ in North India. Nurse Radha _______ Hindi fluently. (speak)
6. There are reports in the newspaper about a seven-year-old child _______ by a mad dog. A mad dog _______ the child. (bite)
7. Has the bell _______? I will _______ the bell tomorrow. (ring)
8. A researcher _______ a detailed investigation. The research was _______ by Dr. Preeti Singhania. (conduct)
9. They _______ all the way to Everest Base Camp. (trek)
10. She _______ ten hours daily to prepare for her goal. She has _______ the Palk Strait last year. (swim)

Here is a list of the present tense, past tense and past participle form of verbs. Remember that the list includes strong verbs, weak verbs, regular verbs and irregular verbs. In some grammar books, you may come across a similar list but titled as regular and irregular verbs. Do not get confused. The lists are the same.

| **Present tense** | **Past tense** | **Past participle** |
|---|---|---|
| abide | Abode | abode |
| arise | arose | arisen |

| Present tense | Past tense | Past participle |
|---|---|---|
| bear (bring forth) | bore | born |
| bear (carry) | bore | borne |
| beat | beat | beaten |
| become | became | become |
| beget | begot | begotten |
| begin | began | begun |
| behold | beheld | beheld |
| bid | bid, bade | bid, bade |
| bind | bound | bound |
| bite | bit | bitten |
| blow | blew | blown |
| break | broke | broken |
| chide | chid | chidden, chid |
| choose | chose | chosen |
| cleave (split) | clove | cloven |
| cling | clung | clung |
| come | came | come |
| dig | dug | dug |
| do | did | done |
| draw | drew | drawn |
| drink | drank | drunk |
| drive | drove | driven |
| eat | ate | eaten |
| fall | fell | fallen |
| fight | fought | fought |

| Present tense | Past tense | Past participle |
|---|---|---|
| find | found | found |
| fling | flung | flung |
| fly | flew | flown |
| forbear | forbore | forborne |
| forbid | forbade | forbidden |
| forget | forgot | forgotten |
| forsake | forsook | forsaken |
| freeze | froze | frozen |
| get | got | got |
| give | gave | given |
| go | went | gone |
| grind | ground | ground |
| grow | grew | grown |
| hide | hid | hidden |
| hold | held | held |
| know | knew | known |
| lie (recline) | lay | lain |
| ride | rode | ridden |
| ring | rang | rung |
| rise | rose | risen |
| run | ran | run |
| see | saw | seen |
| shake | shook | shaken |
| shine | shone | shone |
| shoot | shot | shot |

| Present tense | Past tense | Past participle |
|---|---|---|
| shrink | shrank | shrunk |
| sing | sang | sung |
| sink | sank | sunk |
| sit | sat | sat |
| slay | slew | slain |
| slide | slid | slid |
| sling | slung | slung |
| slink | slunk | slunk |
| smite | smote | smitten |
| speak | spoke | spoken |
| spin | spun | spun |
| spring | sprang | sprung |
| stand | stood | stood |
| steal | Stole | Stolen |
| stick | stuck | stuck |
| sting | stung | stung |
| stink | stunk | stunk |
| stride | strode | stridden |
| strike | struck | struck |
| string | strung | strung |
| strive | strove | striven |
| swear | swore | sworn |
| swim | swam | swum |
| swing | swung | swung |
| take | took | taken |

| Present tense | Past tense | Past participle |
|---|---|---|
| tear | tore | torn |
| throw | threw | thrown |
| tread | trod | trodden, trod |
| wear | wore | worn |
| weave | wove | woven |
| win | won | won |
| wind | wound | wound |
| wring | wrung | wrung |
| write | wrote | written |
| bereave | bereft | bereft |
| beseech | besought | besought |
| bleed | bled | bled |
| breed | bred | bred |
| bring | brought | brought |
| build | built | built |
| burn | burnt | burnt |
| buy | bought | bought |
| catch | caught | caught |
| creep | crept | crept |
| deal | dealt | dealt |
| dwell | dwelt | dwelt |
| feed | fed | fed |
| feel | felt | felt |
| flee | fled | fled |
| have | had | had |

| Present tense | Past tense | Past participle |
|---|---|---|
| keep | kept | kept |
| kneel | knelt | knelt |
| lay | laid | laid |
| lead | led | led |
| learn | learnt | learnt |
| leave | left | left |
| lend | lent | lent |
| lose | lost | lost |
| make | made | made |
| mean | meant | meant |
| meet | met | met |
| pay | paid | paid |
| say | said | said |
| seek | sought | sought |
| sell | sold | sold |
| send | sent | sent |
| shoe | shod | shod |
| sleep | slept | slept |
| smell | smelt | smelt |
| spell | spelt | spelt |
| spend | spent | spent |
| sweep | swept | swept |
| teach | taught | taught |
| Tell | told | told |
| think | thought | thought |

| Present tense | Past tense | Past participle |
|---|---|---|
| weep | wept | wept |
| burst | burst | burst |
| cast | cast | cast |
| cost | cost | cost |
| cut | cut | cut |
| hit | hit | hit |
| hurt | hurt | hurt |
| let | let | let |
| put | put | put |
| read | read | read |
| rid | rid | rid |
| set | set | set |
| shed | shed | shed |
| shut | shut | shut |
| slit | slit | slit |
| split | split | split |
| spread | spread | spread |
| thrust | thrust | thrust |
| wed | wed | wed |
| awake | awoke (awaked) | awoken (awaked) |
| crow | crew (crowed) | crowed |
| hang | hung (hanged) | hung (hanged) |
| thrive | throve (thrived) | thriven (thrived) |
| wake | woke (waked) | woken (waked) |

## AUXILIARIES

We now come to the last aspect of verbs – Auxiliary verbs. By this time you have got your doubts reduced/cleared regarding gerunds, participles, tenses and infinitives. We will now concentrate on the words which work as secondary verbs or helping verbs.

Verbs in any language are quite complex. It is the same in English too. Many books these days give different methods of classifying verbs. Do not get confused. They all finally teach you or show you how the language works. According to recent linguistic studies, verbs may be classified into *lexical and auxiliary* verbs. **Lexical verbs** are words bearing meaning (meaning-bearing)-they carry the meaning of action.

There are verbs which act as helpers. They help the above mentioned lexical verbs to express tense, voice, interrogation and negation. They are called as **auxiliary verbs**.



Let us see a few examples of both lexical verbs and auxiliary verbs.

1. Sita *sang* the prayer melodiously.
2. The boys *cheered* with gusto.
3. I like *swimming* in the sea.
4. The surgeon *spoke* softly.

Here *sang, cheered, swimming, spoke* are lexical verbs or yes just verbs as they show action.

i. The students *were* talking loudly.
ii. I *have* eaten the cake.
iii. What *does* a surgeon do to relax after a lengthy operation?
iv. We *don't* have a digital camera.

Here *were, have, does, don't* are auxiliary verbs. They do not have meanings all by themselves. Their presence helps us to understand the time (of the action) we are talking about (in other words tenses), when we are using the passive voice and whether we are asking questions or expressing a negation.

> ***Note #1:*** Auxiliaries are also called Anomalous or Special verbs or Helping verbs in some books.
>
> ***Note #2:*** Auxiliaries are the only verbs that can make question forms; can combine with *-n't* in the negative (ex: *isn't, haven't*) and can serve to make question tags (ex: *'isn't it?', 'can't you?'*) or stand for a whole verb group in appended statements. (Ex: 'She likes spicy snacks, and so do I').

Auxiliary verbs are of three types:

1. Tense auxiliaries
2. 'do' auxiliaries and
3. Modal auxiliaries

Let us know these auxiliaries.

## Tense Auxiliaries

As the name implies, these are used to form tenses. There are chiefly two auxiliaries under this. They are 'Be' and 'Have'.



**Be**

This auxiliary is used:

1. in the formation of the continuous tenses.

   *Example:* She *is* singing.

   I *am* going home.

   He *was* reading.

2. in the formation of the passive.

   *Example:* The door *was* closed.

*Be* followed by the infinitive is used:

i. to show a plan, arrangement or agreement.

   *Example:* I *am* to see her this evening.

   We *are* to be married next month.

ii. to denote command.

   *Example:* You *are* to write your register number in the box given on the first page of your booklet.

   Father says you *are* to go to college today.

iii. in the past tense with the perfect infinitive to show an arrangement that was made but not carried out.

*Example:* They *were* to have their exam last month but the university had to postpone the exam until the first week of June due to the elections.

***Note #1:*** Present participle form is 'being' and the past participle form is 'been'.

***Note #2:*** The change of tense from present to past to future is seen only in the auxiliary verb and not in the lexical verb.

Here is a table to help you with this auxiliary and the tense forms.

| Pronoun | Present Tense | | Past Tense | | Future Tense | |
|---|---|---|---|---|---|---|
| | Singular | Plural | Singular | Plural | Singular | Plural |
| First person | I am | We are | I was | We were | I shall be | We shall be |
| Second person | You are | You are | You were | You were | You will be | You will be |
| Third person | He/she/it is | They are | He/she/it was | They were | He/she/it will be | They will be |



**Have**

This has only two forms in the present tense – '*has*' and '*have*'. One form only in the past tense for all persons and numbers- '*had*'. In the present participle form – 'having' and past participle form '*had*'.

1. This auxiliary is used in the formation of the perfect tense.

   *Example:* She *has* written the letter.

   He *has* been working.

2. It is used with the infinitive to indicate obligation like,

   I *have* to be there by three o' clock.

   She *has* to cook for herself.

There are two ways of using *have*. They are:

1. Anomalous form (used without do, does, did in negatives and questions).
2. Non-anomalous form (used with do, does, did).

The anomalous form is used when the reference is to a particular occasion. The non-anomalous form is often used with reference to a habitual or permanent state. Like,

i. *Have* you to go early tomorrow to office? (Particular occasion)

   Do you *have* to go early to office? (Habitually, as a rule).

ii. I *haven't* to go to college today.

   I don't *have* to go to college on Sundays.

Here is a table to help you with the tense forms.

| Pronoun | Present Tense |
|---|---|
| I/we/you/they | Have |
| He/she/it | has |

| Perfect Tense | Auxiliary Form |
|---|---|
| Present | Has/have |
| Past | Had |
| Future | Shall/will have |

## 'do' auxiliaries

1. This is used to form the negative and interrogative of the present simple and past simple tenses of non-anomalous verbs. Like,

   He *doesn't* swim. He *didn't* swim.

   *Does* she read? *Did* she write?

2. This auxiliary is used to avoid repetition of a previous ordinary (non-anomalous) verb. Like,

   *Do* you know them? Yes. I *do*.

   He writes well. Yes. He *does*.

   You met her, *didn't* you?

   She sings well and so *do* you.

3. This is also used to emphasize the affirmative nature of a statement.

   *Example:* You *do* look tired.

   I told her not to go, but she *did* go.

4. In an imperative sentence, do makes a request or invitation more persuasive. Like,

   *Do* come back quickly.

   Oh, *do* come! It's an exciting trip.

   In such cases do is strongly stressed.

**Note:** *Doesn't, don't, didn't* are the shortened forms of 'does not', 'do not' and 'did not'. We usually use the shortened forms when we speak.



## Modal auxiliary

These are verbs which when combined with a lexical verb modify their meaning by giving ideas like permission, possibility, obligation or necessity.

*Example:* *May* I sit down? Yes. You may. (Permission)

You *should* obey your parents. (Obligation)

We *must* educate ourselves. (Necessity)

Modals help in communication.

The commonly used modal auxiliaries are:

| | | | |
|---|---|---|---|
| can | shall | must | used |
| could | should | ought | |
| may | will | need | |
| might | would | dare | |

These are divided into **paired forms** and **single forms**.

| Paired forms | Single forms |
|---|---|
| 1. can, could | must |
| 2. may, might | ought |
| 3. shall, should | need |
| 4. will, would | dare |
| | used |

## Can, could

1. *Can* usually expresses ability or capacity. Like,

   I *can* embroider a dress.

   She *can* work these algebraic sums.

   *Can* you lift this trunk?

2. *Can* is used in interrogative and negative sentences.

   *Example:* *Can* this be true?

   She *cannot* refuse this offer.

3. *Could* is used as the past equivalent of can. Like,

   I *could* dance till morning when I was young. (Ability)

   He wondered whether it *could* happen. (Possibility)

4. These days *could* is used as a less positive version of *can*.

   *Example:* I *could* attend the function.

   *Could* you pass me the salt? (Polite request)

## May, might

1. *May* is used to express permission.

   *Example:* You *may* go now.

   *May* I borrow your pencil?

**Note:** Most Asians use *can* while asking permission. This is incorrect as *can* denotes ability. Like,

*Can* I go now? × Here *can* shows that the person has the ability to move from one place to another So the question is misplaced.

*May* I go now? This asks permission.

2. *May* is used to express possibility in affirmative sentences.

*Example:* It *may* rain tomorrow.

She *may* be in the library.

**Note:** Compare 'It *cannot* be true' with 'It *may not* be true'.

*Cannot* denotes impossibility. *May not* denotes improbability.



3. In formal English *may* is used to express a wish.

*Example: May* you live long and happy!

4. *Might* is used as the past equivalent of *May*.

*Example:* She said I *might* write that letter. (Permission)

I thought they *might* be at home. (Possibility)

5. *Might* is used to express a degree of dissatisfaction or reproach.

*Example:* You *might* pay a little more attention to your dress.

## Shall, should, will, would

1. *Shall* is used in the first person and *will* in the second and third person to express pure future.

*Example:* I *shall* be fifty next birthday.

When *shall* we meet again?

Tomorrow *will* be very busy.

You *will* see that I am right.

In present day English, there is a growing tendency to use *will* in all persons.

2. *Shall* is used in the first and third person to ask after the will of the person addressed.

   *Example:* *Shall* I open the door?

   Which pen *shall* I buy?

   *Shall* the waiter serve lunch now?

3. *Will* is used to show

   i. Volition. Like,

   I *will* carry your books. (am willing)

   She *will* do better next time. (Promise to)

   ii. Characteristic habit. Like,

   She *will* talk about nothing but her son.

   He *will* sit for hours reading chemistry.

   iii. Assumption or probability. Like,

   This *will* be the CD you want, I suppose.

   That *will* be the delivery boy, I think.

   iv. '*Will* you?' indicates an invitation or a request. Like,

   *Will* you have coffee?

   *Will* you lend me some money?

   v. *Should* and *Would* are used as the past equivalents of *shall* and *will*.

   *Example:* I expected that I *would* win the race.

   She *should* have finished her education by now.

   vi. *Should* is used in all persons to express duty or obligation.

   *Example:* All *should* obey the laws.

   One *should* keep one's promise.

   Children *should* learn good manners.

vii. In clauses of condition, *should* is used to express a supposition that may not be true.

*Example:* If it *should* rain, the party will be cancelled.

If she *should* see him here, she will be irritated.

viii. *Should* and *would* are also used to show want, polite request, past obligation, probability and a strong desire.

*Example:* I *should* like you to assist her today. (polite form of want)

*Would* you lend me your book, please? ('*Would* you?' is more polite than '*Will* you?')

[Polite request]

You *should* have studied hard. (A past obligation)

She *should* be in the surgery now. (Probability)

I wish he *would* come quickly. (A strong desire)



## Must, Ought

1. *Must* expresses necessity or obligation.

*Example:* We *must* obey the traffic rules.

One *must* work hard to succeed in life.

2. *Must* shows fixed determination. Like,

I *must* get the first rank this year.

She *must* be thirty-seven by now.

3. *Ought* (to) is used to show moral obligation or desirability.

*Example:* We *ought* to be friendly with neighbours.

They *ought* to help him.

4. *Ought* may sometimes express strong probability.

*Example:* Naina *ought* to be helpful.

The show *ought* to be a success.

## Used (to), Need, Dare

1. The auxiliary verb *used* (to) shows a discontinued habit.

   *Example:* There *used* to be a bungalow there.

   I *used* to live in that colony when I was a little girl.

2. *Need* shows necessity or obligation. It is used with the infinitive to form negative and interrogative sentences.

   *Example:* She need not come. (It is not necessary for her to come)

   Need I write to her?

   They hardly need our assistance.

3. When *need* is conjugated with 'do', it has the forms needs, needed and is used with a to- infinitive. It is usually used in negatives and questions. It sometimes occurs in the affirmative too.

   *Example:* Do you *need* to leave now?

   You don't *need* to meet them.

   One *needs* to be careful on wet floors.

4. The auxiliary dare (means be brave enough to) is distinct from the ordinary verb dare(means challenge). It is generally used in negative and interrogative sentences. It takes an infinitive when used with 'do'.

   *Example:* She *dares* (to) talk here. (Affirmative)

   You *dare* not wear the T-shirt today. (Negative)

   How dare you disobey me? (Interrogative)

   She *doesn't dare* to speak to the Principal.

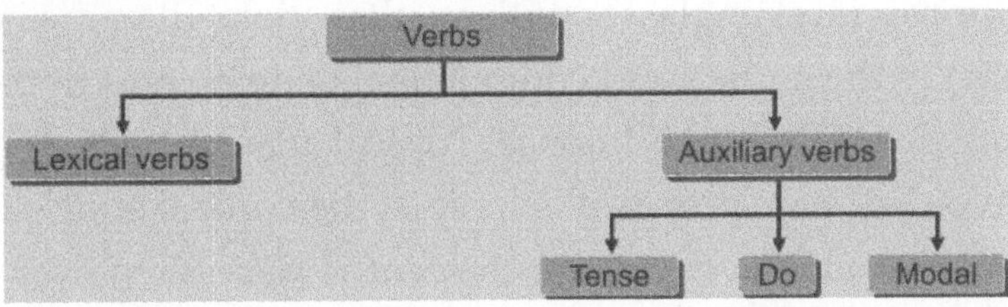

## Exercises

**I. Choose the correct alternatives:**

1. I don't think he (shall, should, can) be able to lift it.
2. She (shall, will, dare) not pay unless she is compelled.
3. You (should, would, ought) be punctual.
4. I wish you (should, would, must) tell m earlier.
5. (Shall, will, would) I assist him?
6. She said I (can, might, may) use her telephone at anytime.
7. If you (shall, should, would) see them, give them my wishes.
8. He (need, dare, would) not ask for a promotion, for fear of losing his job.
9. I (needn't to see, needn't have seen, didn't need to see) her, so I sent a letter.
10. She (am to leave, would leave, was to have left) on Saturday. But on Saturday she had fever, so she decided to wait till Wednesday.
11. He (used, is used, was used) to play hockey before his marriage.
12. He (shall, will, dare) sit outside his garden gate for hours at a time, looking at the passing traffic.
13. '(Might, could, should) she come with us to the drama?'
14. (Might, must, will) I have a glass of water?
15. 'You (ought, will, can) go slow on sugar,' said Dr.Suresh.

**II. This is an extract on Snow blindness in high altitudes. Fill in the blanks with the appropriate auxiliaries:**

In snowscapes reflected sun ______ be very intense. This ________ result in snow blindness up to four hours after exposure if appropriate sunglasses with an ultra-violet filter are not worn. Snowblindness is solar damage (sunburn) to the cornea and conjunctival oedema and hyperaemia, and ______ not appear until the following day. The pain is intense. Topical anaesthetic _____ be used to examine the eye but __________ be avoided thereafter as it is toxic to the corneal epithelium and _______ reduce awareness of further trauma. However, where descent is necessary over difficult terrain topical anaesthetics _____ be required. Treatment consists of oral analgesia (non-steroidal anti-inflammatory drugs __________ be tried first), topical lubricant (e.g. 1% chloramphenicol), eye pads and a cycloplegic (1% cyclopentolate). Healing typically occurs over two to three days.

**III. Here are two sets of instructions given to people learning quilting. Fill in the blanks with the appropriate modals from the choice given in the box at the end:**

**First set of instructions:**

The appliqué background ________ be either a light or dark fabric. It ________ be solid or printed. You ______ be able to create a variety of effects by varying your fabric combination. To test the overall impact of your fabric, cut one spoke from each of the spoke fabrics and arrange them on your appliqué background. If any one spoke matches the background too closely in colour or scale, it ______ be eliminated. A nice balance _________ exist between the plates and the appliqué background. Even if the appliqué background is a dark printed fabric, the plate _____ and ________ be the focal point.

| Can, may, will, should |
|---|

**Second set of instructions:**

The same basic steps __________ be followed to join rows together. Join rows #1 and #2, then #3 and #4, and then #2 and #3. This order __________ keep the bulk of the quilt off your lap for the longest possible time.

Consistency _____________ be maintained to keep the seams in the backing regular. For example, if rows #1 and #2 are being prepared for seaming in the backing, the bottom of the quilt _____________ be near your body, the top of the quilt extending away from you. Right side down, row #1 _________ be on the right and row #2 __________ be on the left. As the left seam allowance is pinned over the right, it __________ be possible to line up the backing seams between the blocks. As you bind stitch, secure any gaps that were not stitched as blocks were joined and any loose seams where threads were accidently clipped.

We come to the end of Verbs. Go slow whenever you have doubts. Read and re-read to get a point clear. When you do this, there is no chance that you will go wrong.

Let us now move to another interesting chapter, All about Adverbs.

Chapter 8

# All About Adverbs

Look at these sentences:

1. Nurse Padma runs.

   Nurse Padma runs quickly.

2. This is a cute child.

   This is a very cute child.

3. Student nurse Laxman reads clearly.

   Student nurse Laxman reads quite clearly.

In the first sentence, *quickly* shows how (or in what manner) Padma runs; that is, *quickly* modifies the verb *runs*.

In the second sentence, *very* shows how much (or in what degree) the child is cute; that is, very modifies the adjective *cute*.

In the third sentence, *quite* shows how far (or to what extent) Laxman reads *clearly*; that is, *quite* modifies the adverb *clearly*.

*Definition:* An adverb is a word which modifies (or adds more to) the meaning of a verb, an adjective or another adverb.

## Exercises

**I. Underline the adverbs in these sentences:**

1. He smiled happily.
2. She is seriously ill.
3. I wasn't slightly surprised with the outcome.

4. Fortunately, nobody was injured.
5. My younger brother sings awfully.
6. The old man drove rashly.
7. The short man spoke quietly and calmly.
8. It rained sporadically.

**II. Correct these sentences:**

1. She drove slow.
2. He was real glad to see her.
3. He beat us easy.
4. She spoke to him as calm as possible
5. The doctor diagnosed correct.
6. Ward boys walked quick.
7. Senior surgeon Vasudev Rao talks rapid.
8. The wards are cleaned vigorous.

## Kinds of Adverb

**Adverbs are divided into 7 kinds according to the meaning/use. They are :**

i. Adverbs of Time
ii. Adverbs of Frequency
iii. Adverbs of Place
iv. Adverbs of Manner
v. Adverbs of Degree or Quantity
vi. Adverbs of Affirmation and Negation
vii. Adverbs of Reason

## Adverbs of Time

These are words which show *when* the action (verb) has taken place.

*Example:*

1. She has heard this *before*.
2. The doctors have seen this *before*.
3. The ward boys were here a few minutes *ago*.
4. The end *soon* came.
5. Nurses report to the nursing station *daily*.



## Adverbs of Frequency

These are words which show *how often* the action has taken place.

*Example:*

1. The wife repeated the instruction *twice*.
2. The trekker experienced *hypoxia* whenever he had to climb along with his heavy backpack.
3. The students often make mistakes.
4. The Resident surgeon seldom visits this block.

## Adverbs of Place

These are words which show *where* the action is taking place.

*Example:*

1. Is the Doctor *in*?
2. The doctor asked the patient to walk *backward*.
3. "*Sit here*", ordered the teacher.
4. The dogs ran *away*.

## Adverbs of Manner

These are words which show *how* or *in what manner* the action is carried out.

*Example:*

1. Student nurse Laxman reads *clearly*.
2. This report is *well* written.
3. The child slept *soundly*.
4. The soldiers fought *bravely*.

> ***Note:*** This Adverb includes nearly all words which are derived from Adjectives and end in '- ly.'

## Adverbs of Degree or Quantity

These are words which show *how much* or in what degree or to what extent the action is.

*Example:*

1. The patient was *too* careless with the reports.
2. These fruits are *almost* ripe.
3. The weather is *very* stormy.
4. The condition of the patient in bed 18 is *no* better today.

## Adverbs of Affirmation and Negation

These are words which show *whether the action has taken place or not.*

*Example:*

1. The diabetic in the men's ward *certainly* went home.
2. *Surely* you are mistaken.
3. He *does not* know me.

## *Adverbs of Reason*

These are words which analyse the cause of the action.

*Example:*

1. Ruskin's parents died. There is no one to pay his fees. He *therefore* left medical college.

   Some adverbs may belong to more than one class, like–

2. They went *far*. (Adverb of Place)
3. The patient is *far* better now. (Adverb of Degree)
4. He sings *delightfully*. (Adverb of Manner)
5. The weather is *delightfully* cool. (Adverb of Degree)

## Exercise



**Underline the adverbs and identify the class that they belong to:**

1. She was ill pleased. ____________________
2. Try, try, try again till you succeed. ________________
3. She is too shy to go into the men's ward. ________________
4. Too many cooks spoil the broth. ________________
5. Grand-father is somewhat better. ________________
6. She went off on Monday. ________________
7. His health is no worse than before. ________________
8. The operation theater is ready. The doctors will now begin the surgery. ____________________
9. I hurt my elbow the day before yesterday. ________________
10. The professor called again. ____________________
11. The Medical Director formerly lived in this bungalow. ________________
12. The patient complained frequently of nausea. ____________________
13. The little child followed it's mother everywhere. ____________________
14. The nurses have not seen that complaining boy even once. ____________________
15. My sister is out. ____________________

16. The hospitals must always be efficient. ____________

17. The guests were very kindly received. ____________

18. The mountain doctors in the Himalayas often do house visits on skis. ____________

19. The student doctor was quite wrong in his analysis. ____________

20. I do not agree with him. ____________

Some words are used sometimes as adjectives and sometimes as adverbs like:

| Adjectives | Adverbs |
|---|---|
| The patient spoke in a *loud* voice. | He talks so *loud*. |
| He is a *fast* bowler. | He can bowl *fast*. |
| The doctor lives in the *next* house. | The *next* time she saw him, she decided to speak to him. |
| They crowded at the *back* entrance. | Go *back*. |
| That was a *hard* sum. | The surgeon works *hard* all day. |
| The old man is *quick* to take offence. | Run *quick*. |
| Is he an *early* riser? | They started *early*. |
| She is the *only* child of his parents. | You can *only* guess. |

*Always remember:* Only by noticing *how* a word is used, that we can tell what part of speech it is.

Use the words given below in sentences of your own (1) as Adjectives (2) as Adverbs:

Very, near, ill, only, clean, long, late, early, fast

## Comparison of Adverbs

Like adjectives, some adverbs have three degrees of comparison.

1. If the adverb is of one syllable, comparative degree is formed by adding '-er' at the end. The superlative is formed by adding '-est' to the positive.
2. Adverbs that end in 'ly' form the comparative by adding *more* and the superlative by adding '*most*'.
3. Some form the comparative and superlative degree irregularly:

| Positive | Comparative | Superlative |
|---|---|---|
| Fast | Faster | Fastest |
| Long | Longer | Longest |
| Hard | Harder | Hardest |
| Soon | Sooner | Soonest |
| Swiftly | More swiftly | Most swiftly |
| Skillfully | More skillfully | Most skillfully |

| | | |
|---|---|---|
| Early | Earlier | Earliest |
| Ill, badly | Worse | Worst |
| Well | Better | Best |
| Much | More | Most |
| Little | Less | Least |
| Nigh, Near | Nearer | Next |
| Far | Farther/ Further | Farthest/ Furthest |
| Late | Later | Last |

*Note:* • Only adverbs of manner, degree and time can have degrees of comparison.
• Many adverbs do not have degrees of comparison

*Example:* Now, then, there, once.

Write the three degrees of comparison for these adverbs:
Suddenly, often, near, loud, hard, wisely, patiently.

| Positive | Comparative | Superlative |
|---|---|---|
| | | |

## Formation of Adverbs

- Adverbs of Manner are mostly formed from adjectives by adding 'ly'

*Example:*

| **Adjective** | **Adverbs of Manner** |
|---|---|
| Clever | Cleverly |
| Wise | Wisely |

| | |
|---|---|
| Kind | Kindly |
| Foolish | Foolishly |
| Quick | Quickly |
| Beautiful | Beautifully |

*Example Sentences:*

1. Solomon was a wise king.
2. He ruled wisely for many years.

- When the adjective ends in 'y' and has a consonant before it, y changes to 'i' and 'ly' is added.

*Example:*

| **Adjective** | **Adverb** |
|---|---|
| Happy | Happily |
| Ready | Readily |
| Heavy | Heavily |

- Exceptions (which do not follow this rule) are:

| **Adjective** | **Adverb** |
|---|---|
| Shy | Shyly |
| Sly | Slyly |
| Dry | Dryly |

- If the adjective ends in 'le', 'e' is changed into 'y'

*Example:*

| **Adjective** | **Adverb** |
|---|---|
| Single | Singly |
| Double | Doubly |

- If the adjective ends in 'l', 'ly' is added. Ending becomes 'lly'

*Example:*

| **Adjective** | **Adverb** |
|---|---|
| Real | Really |
| Careful | Carefully |

- If the adjective ends in 'e', 'e' is retained and 'ly' is added.

*Example:*

| **Adjective** | **Adverb** |
|---|---|
| Safe | Safely |
| Nice | Nicely |
| Extreme | Extremely |

- There are exceptions to this rule:

| **Adjective** | **Adverb** |
|---|---|
| True | Truly |
| Due | Duly |
| Whole | Wholly |

- If an adjective ends in 'ic', only 'lly' is added

*Example:*

| **Adjective** | **Adverb** |
|---|---|
| Automatic | Automatically |
| Basic | Basically |

Exception to this is public publicly

- Some adverbs are made up of a noun and a qualifying adjective.

  *Example:* Sometimes, meantime, meanwhile, yesterday, midway

- A few adverbs are compounds of 'on' (weakened to 'a') and a noun.

  *Example:* a foot (=on foot), abed, asleep, ahead, aboard, away, afar.

- A few adverbs are compounds of a Preposition and an Adjective.

  *Example:* a long, aloud, anew, behind, below, beyond.

- A few Adverbs are compounds of a Preposition and an Adverb.

  *Example:* within, without, before, beneath.

- Some Adverbs are formed when two Adverbs are joined together by a Conjunction.

*Like:*

again and again (= repeatedly)

by and by (= after a time).

far and near (= in all directions)

far and wide (= everywhere)

far and away (=by a great deal)

first and foremost (= first of all)

now and then (= occasionally)

now and again (=Sometimes)

off and on (= not regularly)

out and out (= beyond all comparison)

over and over (=frequently)

through and through (= completely)

to and fro (= backwards and forwards)

By this time a few of you will be confused about using these in sentences. Relax. It is easy. Listen to people talking around you. You can recognize many more adverbs.

*Example:*

1. Read good books *again and again.*
2. The doctor warned the obese patient *again and again* to reduce his food intake.
3. *By and by* all the babies settled down in the crèche.
4. Her fame has spread *far and near.*
5. As a medical administrator he saw *far and wide.*
6. Doctor Rao is *far and away* the best Orthopedic Surgeon.
7. Once the baby is born, the *first and foremost* work is to clean it.
8. I write to my parents *now and then.*
9. She worked for fifteen years, *off and on* in the nursing department of our hospital.
10. The students believed their pathology notes were *out and out* the best.
11. Children read all the Harry Potter books *over and over.*
12. I have read the Bible *through and through.*
13. Men whose wives are delivering their babies walk *to and fro* outside the labour room.



## Exercises

**I. Form adverbs from the words given:**

quick ______________ incredible ______________

steady ______________ terrible ______________

lucky ______________ gentle ______________

merry ______________ idle ______________

temporary ___________ easy ______________

**II. Complete the sentences with adverbs:**

1. We didn't go to college because it was raining ______________.
2. Their team lost the game because they played very ______________.

3. The patients had to wait for a long time, but they didn't complain. They waited ______________.
4. The emergency room nurses keep fit by doing yoga ______________.
5. The pillion rider on the scooter was ______________ injured in the accident.

**III. Fill in the blanks with the correct Adverb given in the bracket:**

1. The ambulance was forced to move ____________ due to a massive traffic jam. (slowly/fastly)
2. The doctor advised my neighbour to take her medication for diabetes______________. (regularly/again and again)
3. The lamp lighting ceremony will start ____________ .(immediately/shortly)
4. We should not talk ______________ in a hospital. (softly/loudly)
5. Ward boy Stefan greets all patients _________ in the morning. (cheerfully/slowly)
6. Rajini likes wearing ____________ clothes after her hospital duty is over. (colourful/colourfully)
7. He fell and hurt himself quite _________. (badly/safely)
8. The doctor glared ______________ at his assistant for interrupting him. (angrily/happily)
9. It wasn't a serious accident. The auto was only ____________ damaged. (slightly/unusually)
10. The Casualty Department was ______________ busy today. (unusually/unnecessarily)

You now know how to use Adverbs. Don't forget to practise. Let's move on now.

Chapter 9

# All About Prepositions

Observe these sentences.

1. There is a dog *in* the garden.
2. I am fond *of* tea.
3. The child jumped *off* the chair.

In the first sentence, the word '*in*' shows the relation between two things, *dog* and *garden*.

In the second sentence, the word '*of*' shows the relation between the liking of the taste/drink shown by the adjective *fond* and noun *tea*.

In the third sentence, the word '*off*' shows the relation between the action shown by the verb-*jumped* and the noun-*chair*.

These words are placed either before a noun or a pronoun. Such words are called as **Prepositions.**

***Definition:*** A word which is *placed before* a noun or a pronoun to show in what *relation* the person or thing denoted by it stands in regard to something else is called as a **Preposition**.

Preposition means 'that which is placed before'.

In the first sentence the Preposition joins a Noun to another Noun. In the second it joins a Noun to Adjective and in the third sentence it joins a Noun to a Verb.

## Kinds of Preposition

1. ***Simple prepositions:*** at, by for, from, in, of, off, on, out, through, till, to, up, with.
2. ***Compound prepositions:*** Formed by prefixing a Preposition to a Noun, an Adjective or an Adverb. about, above, across, along, amidst, among, amongst, around, before, behind, below ,beneath, beside, between, beyond, inside, outside, underneath, within, without.

3. ***Phrase prepositions:*** This is a group of words used with the force of a single preposition.

| | | |
|---|---|---|
| according to | in accordance with | in place of |
| agreeably to | in addition to | in reference to |
| along with | on behalf of | in spite of |
| away from | in case of | instead of |
| because of | in comparison to | in the event of |
| by dint of | in consequence of | on account of |
| by means of | in course of | owing to |
| by virtue of | in favour of | with a view to |
| by way of | in front of | with an eye to |
| for the sake of | in order to | with regard to |



## Exercise

**Underline the Prepositions in the sentences given below and name the preposition:**

1. Little Dennis sat in a corner.
2. Humpty Dumpty sat on a wall.
3. The patient in bed 12 requested for some privacy.
4. A cute little girl sat under the table.
5. The labourers work from morning till night.
6. In consequence of her illness she could not finish the work in time.
7. By means of rope ladders they climbed the wall.
8. On behalf of the staff, she gave the speech.
9. The blackboard is behind the teacher.
10. The young girl sitting between the two old people is my cousin.
11. The medical shop is across the street.

12. The nurse looked after the frail old lady according to the instructions given by the doctor.

13. Whatever nurse Linda does, she does with an eye to the main chance.

14. I walked along the beach.

15. They went by the post office.

> **Note:** Several words are used both as Adverbs and as a Preposition. A word is a Preposition if it governs a Noun or Pronoun; it is an Adverb when it does not govern a Noun or Pronoun.

*Example:*

| *Adverb* | *Prepositions* |
|---|---|
| The mother said, "Go and run *about*". | Don't loiter *about* the city. |
| She could not come *before*. | He came the day *before* yesterday. |
| Has the Medical Officer come *in*? | Is he *in* his room? |
| The cap came *off*. | The dog jumped *off* the table. |
| Let them move *on*. | The pens lie *on* the table. |
| Their mothers arrived soon *after*. | *After* a year the patient could walk. |
| Take this *over* to the blood bank. | He rules *over* this vast hospital. |
| The doctor has not seen her *since*. | The nurse has not slept *since* yesterday. |

## Exercises

**I. Choose the correct preposition given in the brackets and fill up the blanks:**

1. This work is ________ the capacity of a student nurse. (beyond/among)
2. It is cool ________ April. (for/to)
3. She was left ________ dead ________ the field. (for, on/in, for)
4. Nothing will come ________ nothing. (in, of)
5. ________ what I know of him, I can't believe he did it. (From/Towards)

6. She charges interest ________ nine percent. (at/which)
7. Cloth is sold ________ the meter. (by/in)
8. ________ his death his children regretted their decisions. (After/In)
9. The students quarrelled ________ themselves. (among/in)
10. The piped piper marched ________ the town. (through/into)
11. The child took medicine ________ a cold. (for/with)
12. Gardens are usually ________ the house. (outside/inside)
13. ________ talking, prove your worth by doing something. (Instead of/Through)
14. ________ her researches Dr. Malini met with many obstacles. (In course of/In case of)
15. ________ Deepavali the educational institutions are closed. (On account of/In favour of)



**II. Fill in the blanks with appropriate prepositions given in the box. A preposition can be repeated as many times as needed:**

| By, of, to, for, in, with, into |
|---|

### Diabetes Mellitus

This common and most dreaded disease is characterized ______ partial inability ______ the body cells ______ use glucose either ______ energy production or glycogen formation. Unused sugar exists ______ the blood and is excreted ______ the urine. The diabetic patient mostly feels very thirsty and hungry and passes frequent and excessive urine. Unable fully ______ utilize sugar ______ energy he loses weight and becomes weak. His blood circulation becomes poor, the blood clots ______ abnormal slowness and minor infections flare up ______ illness. Slow healing ______ wounds may lead ______ tissue death or gangrene. Impaired oxidation ______ glucose also affects metabolism ______ fat. Instead of yielding $CO_2$ and water, fats are changed ______ poisonous acetone (ketone) and ______ acids that may dangerously lower the blood pH and cause ketosis. Diabetics also become prone ______ arteriosclerosis and cataract.

**III. Complete the following passage by filling the blanks with the correct preposition given in the box. Each preposition can be used as many times as required:**

| According to, to, in, from, by, because of, on, for, of, on account of |
|---|

### Kwashiorkor

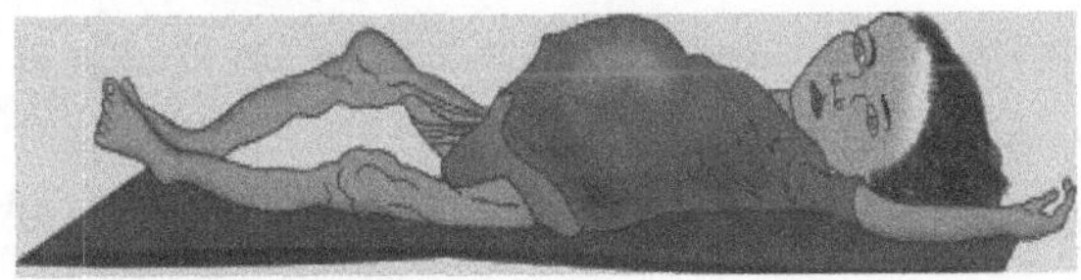

_______________ medical studies, an inadequate protein intake in the diet often leads to protein calorie malnutrition or PCM. PCM is also called protein, energy malnutrition or PEM. One such deficiency is called kwashiorkor.

This disease ______ infants and young children is caused ______ severe protein deficiency. Millions ______ babies ______ Asia including India, Africa and Latin America suffer ______ this deficiency disease. It is caused when instead ______ their mother's milk, they take mainly a carbohydrate diet that too ______ an inadequate amount. The children suffering ______ kwashiorkor become irritable, miserable, cease ______ grow and lose weight. The skin becomes scaly, dark and shows ugly cracks. Hair takes ______ a reddish colour. The body swells ______ water retention ______ the cells (oedema): Belly protrudes and limbs become thin and bony. Brain development and mental capacities are retarded. The liver too is damaged and the child often dies before the age ______ five. Such children also become increasingly susceptible ______ various infections.

On account of poverty ______ Asia and Africa many cases of kwashiorkor are neglected. In the absence ______ mother's milk, a protein-rich diet obtained ______ animals or ______ soya bean, or a mixture ______ corn, cotton-seed, yeast and leaf-meal or a combination ______ wheat, gram, peanuts and jaggery, can effectively cure this African named disease.

**IV. Complete the following passage by filling the blanks with the correct preposition given in the box. Each Preposition can be used as many times as required:**

| According to, to, of, in, without, by, from, for, at, about |
|---|

## Pollution Hazards

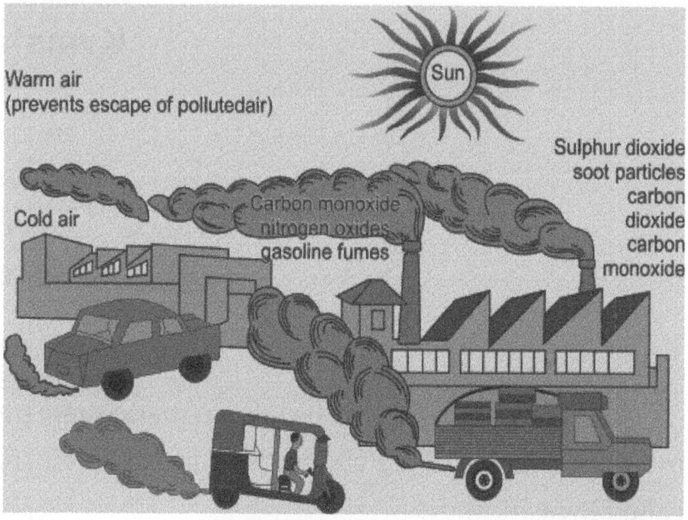

_____________ a report the sulphur dioxide ($SO_2$) content ______ the atmosphere ______ Delhi city has reached the level ______ 0.233 ppm, whereas ______ USA and West Germany the permissible limit is only 0.1 and 0.05 ppm. Concentrations as low as 0.3 ppm may damage plants. Lichens are particularly sensitive to $SO_2$ and ______ polluted regions you do not find lichens growing ______ the tree trunks. Thus, lower quantities ______ sulphur dioxide suppresses the overall vegetative as well as reproductive growth and yield. Its high atmospheric concentrations produce various injuries ______ leaves such as interveinal and blade damage, necrosis ______ leaves and cellular collapse. However, moderate $SO_2$ pollution results ______ chlorosis ______ leaves ______ cellular collapse. Pine trees are more susceptible than broad leaved trees and react ______ partial defoliation and reduced growth. Plant's exposure ______ hydrogen sulphide results ______ leaf lesions, mottling, defoliation and reduced growth.

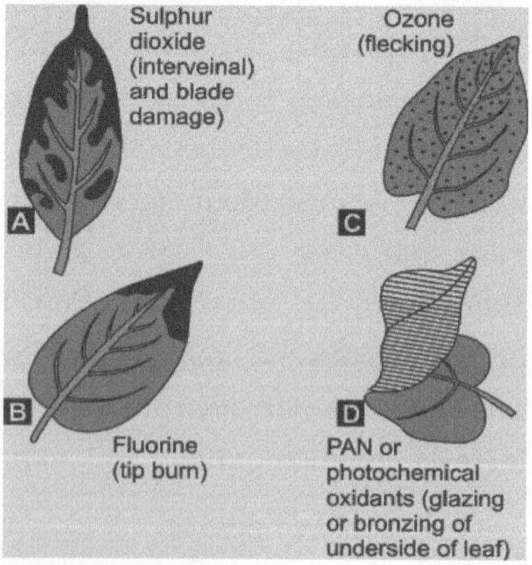

Sulphur dioxide pollution causes ______ human beings various types ______ injuries such as eye irritation, chest constriction, headache, vomiting and death ______ respiratory ailment. It paralyzes or destroys bronchial cilia ______ air passages ______ man, constricts bronchii, damages lungs, lowers resistance ______

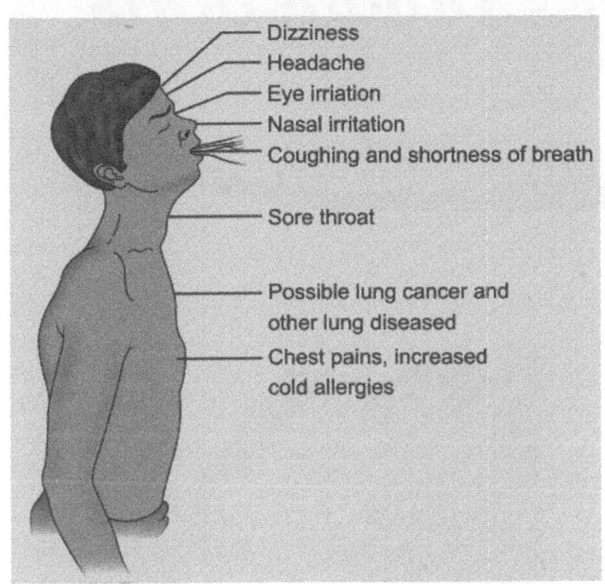


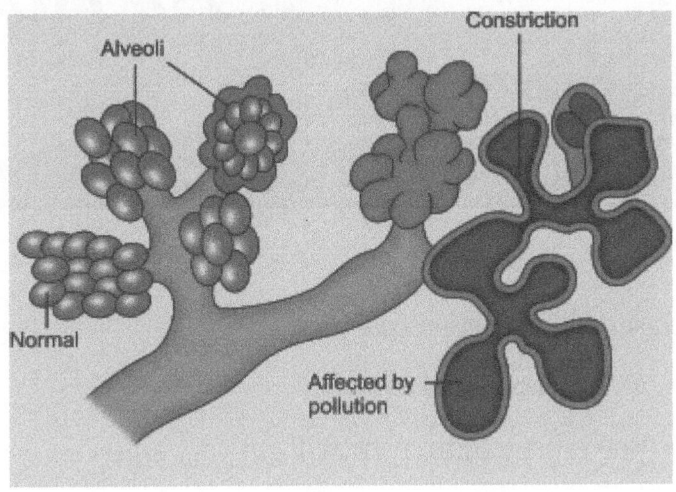


pneumonia and influenza and causes bronchitis, emphysema and irritation ______ the mucous membranes (i.e., an increase ______ cough and sputum). In fact, $SO_2$ and other pollutants bring ______ coalescence ______ alveoli, and reduce the amount ______ surface area available ______ the transport ______ oxygen and also reduce the rate ______ which air is exchanged.

Prepositions are confusing initially. Regular practice helps you in understanding them and using them successfully.

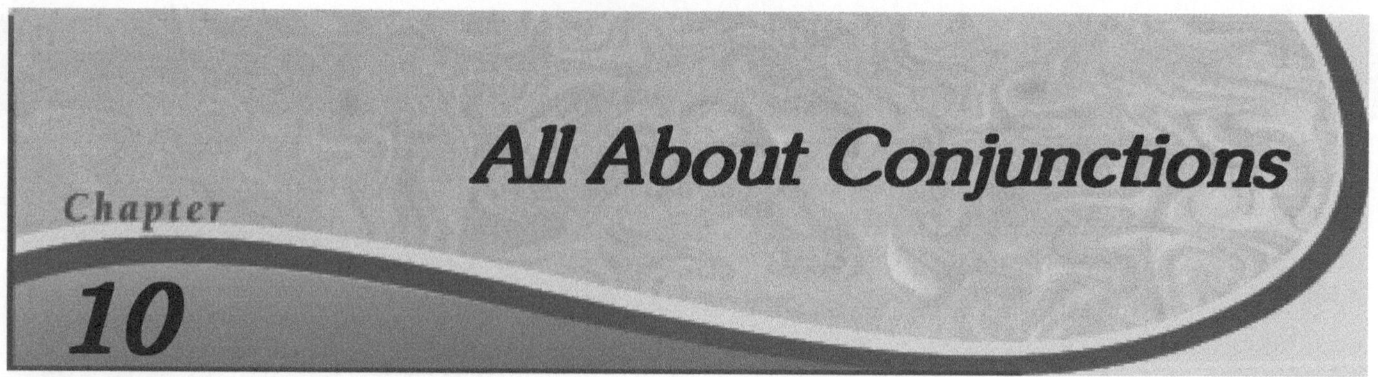


# Chapter 10

# All About Conjunctions

Observe these sentences:

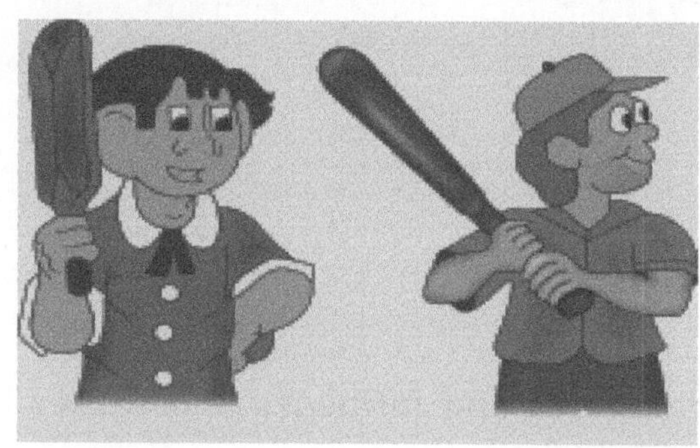

1. One *and* one makes two.
2. She must laugh, *or* she will get very angry.
3. Their wealth is small, *but* their hearts are great.
4. Sachin *and* Dravid are good batsmen.

In these sentences 2, 3, 4 the conjunctions join two sentences together. In sentence 1 it joins two words only.

***Definition:*** A **Conjunction** is a word which joins together sentences and sometimes words and does no other work.

Let us take sentence 3.

Their wealth is small. Their hearts are great.

By writing *but* in between these two sentences we get

Their wealth is small, *but* their hearts are great.

Conjunctions often make the jointed sentences more compact.

***Example:*** Alan is a good bowler and Ahmed is a good bowler.

Instead of such a long sentence, we can write

Alan *and* Ahmed are good bowlers.

**Now, make this sentence compact:**

The man is poor, but he is honest

_______________________________

When conjunctions are used to join words, such sentence cannot be resolved into two sentences.

*Like* Two *and* two makes four.

Aliya *and* Mehnaz are sisters.

> **Note:** Conjunctions should not be confused with Relative Pronouns, Relative Adverbs and Prepositions which are also connecting words.

***Example:***

1. This is the house *that* Roopa built. (Relative Pronouns).
2. This is the spot *where* he was attacked. (Relative Adverb).
3. Take this *and* give that. (Conjunction).

In sentence 1, the Relative Pronoun 'that' *refers to the common noun, house*, and also joins the two parts of a sentence.

This is the house. Roopa built the house.

This is the house *that* Roopa built.

In sentence 2, the Relative Adverb 'where' *modifies the verb was attacked* and also joins the two parts of the sentence.

This is the spot. He was attacked here.

This is the spot *where* he was attacked.

In sentence 3, the Conjunction *and* simply joins the two sentences.

It does no other work.

(You) Take this. Give (me) that.

Take this *and* give that.

So, we can say that relative pronouns and relative adverbs also join sentences; but they do more work.

Conjunctions simply join; they do no other work.

You may now have a doubt regarding preposition as it too joins words. But, it does more.

*Like*

He sat *beside* Rahul. He stood *behind* me.

It takes a little practice to differentiate between Conjunctions and the other grammatical terms that join sentences. Keep practising and you will not have any doubts.

Now some Conjunctions are used in pairs. Like–

1. Either-or
2. Both-and
3. Neither-nor
4. Whether-or
5. Though-yet
6. Not only-but also.



Let us see how these are used in sentences.

1. Either use the purse or give it away.
2. It is neither here nor there.
3. We both love and honour our parents.
4. Though the child is suffering much pain, yet it does not complain.
5. I do not care whether I work here or not.
6. Not only is he stubborn but also stupid.

These conjunctions (used in pairs) are called correlative conjunctions or simply correlatives.

Remember while using correlatives, each of the correlated words should be placed immediately before the words to be connected. Like–

He visited *not only* Kuala Lumpur, *but also* Singapore.

It is not to be written this way–

He not only visited Kaula Lampur, but also Singapore.

**Now try to write six different sentences using the correlatives.**

______________________________________________

______________________________________________

______________________________________________

______________________________________________

______________________________________________

______________________________________________

A few compound expressions are used as conjunctions. They are called compound conjunctions. They are:

in order that, on condition that, even if, so that, provided that, as though, in as much as, as well as, as soon as, as if.

Let us now see how these are used in a sentence.

1. The information was published *in order that* all might know the facts.
2. I will accept the offer *on condition that* the management will provide the required facilities.
3. He saved some water *so that* he need not go thirsty later.
4. You can borrow the stethoscope *provided that* you return it soon.
5. She talks *as though* she is a great traveller.
6. Dr Rao refused the patient's request, *in as much as* he believed it unreasonable.
7. Nurse Ganga *as well as* matron Jane was present there.
8. Dr Brown took off his coat *as soon as* he entered his house.
9. The senior nurse looks *as if* she will faint.

**Try to make sentences on your own now.**

1. ______________________________________________
2. ______________________________________________
3. ______________________________________________

4. ____________________

5. ____________________

6. ____________________

7. ____________________

8. ____________________

9. ____________________

10. ____________________

11. ____________________

Conjunctions are divided into two classes:



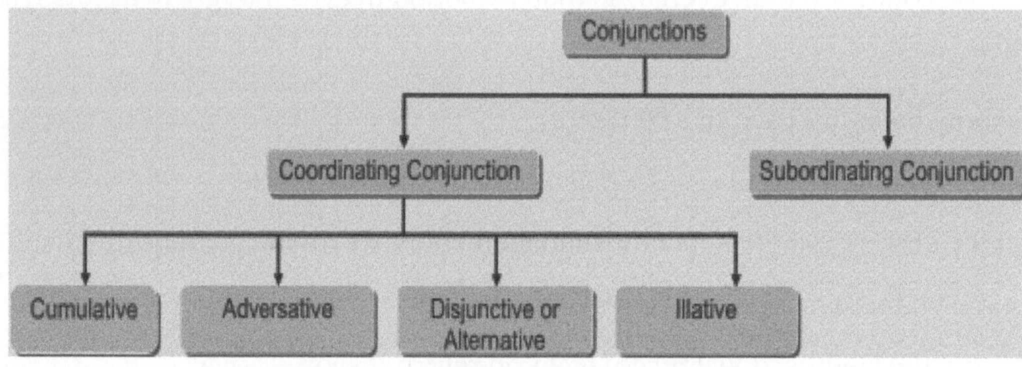


Read this sentence:

Horses run *and* snakes slither.

This has two independent statements or two statements of equal importance.

***Definition:*** Thus, the conjunction joining two statements or clauses of equal importance is called a **Coordinating Conjunction.**

And, but, for, or nor, also, either.....or, neither......nor are Coordinating Conjunctions.

These are of four kinds:

1. ***Cumulative Coordinating Conjunction:*** *These just add one statement to* another. Like–

   Govind bought a T-shirt and guavas today.

2. ***Adversative Coordinating Conjunction:*** *These express the contrast* (opposite) between two statements.
   Like–
   i. She is shy, but she is courageous.
   ii. He was irritated, still he kept quiet.
   iii. They would have come; only that they had to go to the Pooja.
3. ***Disjunctive or Alternative Coordinating Conjunction:*** *These show a choice* between two alternatives.
   Like–
   i. She must laugh, or she will get angry.
   ii. Either he is lame, or he feigns lameness.
   iii. Drive quickly else you will not overtake him.
4. ***Illative Coordinating Conjunction:*** These show inference.
   Like–
   The security must have been lax, for the terrorists got inside the airplane.



## Subordinating Conjunction

Examine these sentences:

1. I read the paper. Reading the paper interests me.

   These two statements can be combined this way by using a conjunction.
2. I read the paper *because* it interests me.

   'because it interests me' is a clause *dependent* on the other part of the statement. Thus, the Conjunction introducing the *dependent or subordinate clause* is called a Subordinating Conjunction.

***Definition:*** A subordinating conjunction is a word which joins a statement or clause to another on which it depends for its full meaning.

After, because, if, that, though, although, till, before, unless, as, when, where, while are the chief subordinating conjunctions.

***Examples:*** *After* the shower was over the patient was put to bed.

1. A cake's a cake, although there is no icing on it.
2. *As* the doctor was not there, I spoke to his assistant.
3. The boys ran away *because* they were afraid of punishment.
4. Answer the matron *before* you proceed further.
5. You will learn good English *if* you work hard.
6. *Since* the Professor Emeritus said so, we must believe it.
7. Inform the class *that* a new professor is handling the class.
8. Svenson finished the exam first *though* he began half an hour late.
9. "You have to wait *till* the doctor returns", said the nurse to the tense mother.
10. Fine will not be paid *unless* it is compelled by law.
11. She waited for her friend *until* she came.
12. *When* my father was a boy, they used silver coins as money.
13. Nurse Rustum found his library card *where* he had left it.
14. The young mother said "I do not understand *how* it all happened" about the accident she saw.
15. Make hay *while* the sun shines.

***Note # 1:*** The word 'than' is also a Subordinating Conjunction.

*Example:*

1. Doctor Raman is taller than Doctor Steve.
2. I like Radiology better *than* Orthopaedics.
3. I like you better *than* her.

Now all these subordinating conjunctions are classified into 7 types according to the meaning they denote:

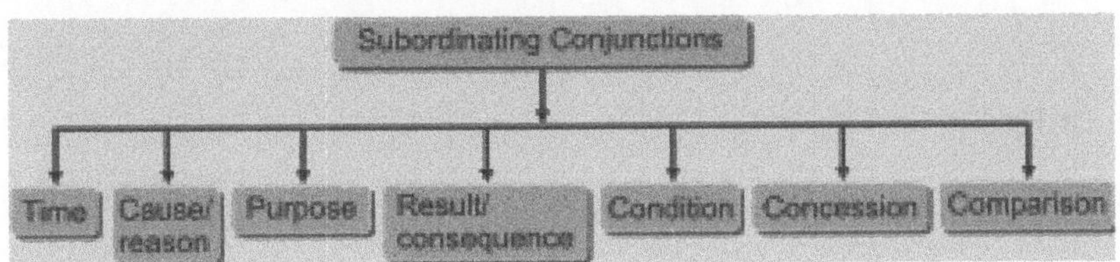


1. ***Let us take Time:***

   Before, till, since, after, once, as soon as, when, while.

   i. The old lady would die *before* she lied.

   ii. *When* Juliane looked at her wounds, she saw maggots crawling over them.

   iii. Many events have taken place *since* I saw you.

   iv. The doctors visited the wards *after* the visiting hours.

2. ***Cause or Reason:***

   Because, since, as, so, so that, as a result, due to, therefore.

   i. Raghav died *because* his tumor could not be removed.

   ii. I took paracetamol tablet yesterday *as I* had fever.

   iii. Our dog Waggy had to be put to sleep *as a result* of kidney failure.

   iv. He may enter the ICU, *as* he is a house surgeon.

3. ***Purpose:***

   That, lest

   i. We drink *that* we may live.

   ii. The nurse held the old man's hand *lest* he should fall.

4. ***Result or Consequence:***

   Nurse Susan was so tired *that* she could scarcely stand.

5. ***Condition:***

If, unless

i. The patient will agree for the surgery, *if* doctor Roshan is the surgeon.

ii. Diseases cannot be cured *unless* they are diagonised properly.

6. ***Concession:***

Though, although

i. A cake's a cake *although* there's no icing on it.

ii. *Though* some patients disobey the doctor, yet they will have to treat them.

7. ***Comparison:***

Matron Roma is stronger than matron Leila [is].



With all this you are confused with similar words in different parts of speech. So let's put your doubts to rest.

Certain words are used both as Prepositions and Conjunctions.

*Example:*

| ***Preposition*** | ***Conjunction*** |
|---|---|
| • Stay *till* Saturday | • Students shall stay here *till* the professor returns. |
| • Soldiers died *for* their country. | • The watchman must stay here, *for* such is his duty. |
| • I have not met the doctor *since* I got well. | • The Nurses shall go to the seminar *since* management desires it. |
| • The cat ran *after* the mouse. | • The patients came *after* the surgeons had left. |
| • Everybody *but* Adam was absent. | • They tried, *but* did not reach the goal. |
| • The students stood *before* the teacher. | • Look *before* you leap. |

Now let us practise using conjunctions.

## Exercises

**I. Underline the conjunction in the following sentences, and state whether they are coordinating or subordinating conjunctions:**

| Sentence | Coordinating Conjunction | Subordinating Conjunction |
|---|---|---|
| 1. They will not succeed unless they work harder. | | |
| 2. The children arrived after the film star had gone. | | |
| 3. Reshma waited till the blood report arrived. | | |
| 4. Fruit and milk is wholesome food. | | |
| 5. A nursing student will get the award if one has worked honestly. | | |
| 6. "When you are called, you must go in at once", the nurse told the patient | | |
| 7. The mother told the child, "Do not go before I come". | | |
| 8. The chemist cannot give any medicine, for he has none. | | |
| 9. Since the Professor Emeritus said so, we must believe it. | | |
| 10. My grandfather is ill, yet he refuses to see a doctor. | | |
| 11. She has to go on an empty stomach since she is going for blood glucose test. | | |
| 12. They performed the CPR but the patient died. | | |
| 13. The service in SAB hospital is neither quick nor efficient. | | |
| 14. Despite the shortage of electric power, the medical staff at the Emergency Wing carried out their work efficiently. | | |
| 15. Dr Ratnam is quicker than Dr Hari. | | |

**II. Fill in the blanks with correct conjunctions:**

1. Be fair_______ fear not.
2. She ran fast, _______ she missed the bus.
3. Do not sit _______ I say so.
4. She finished first _______ she began late.
5. Take a torch, _______ the electricity supply stops.
6. Staff nurse Lalitha is not thorough in her work _______ she is careless.

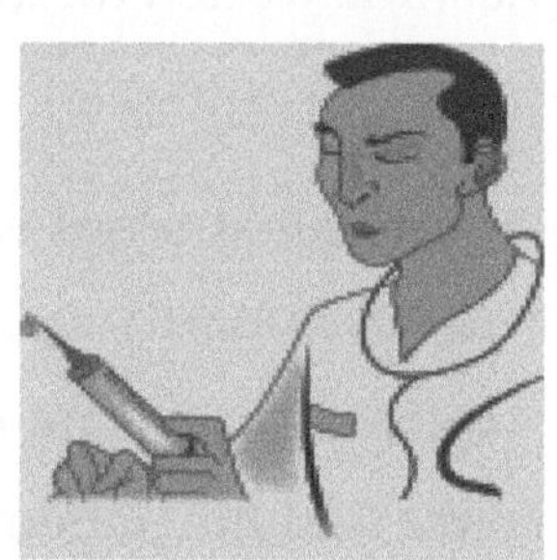

7. The height _______ weight of a person must be proportionate.
8. Good health is staying calm _______ contended.
9. Many children dislike doctors _______ they give injections.
10. I shall not attend the function _______ I have not been invited.
11. _______ duty calls us we must obey.
12. _______ the purse is stolen _______ lost.
13. Seven _______ seven makes fourteen.
14. Is his name Stefan _______ Steven?

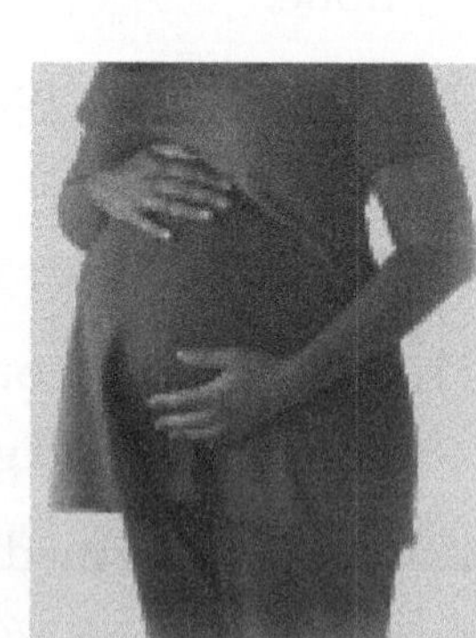

15. They are very rich _______ they are not happy.
16. There is no doubt _______ the woman is pregnant.
17. Water _______ oil will not mix.
18. She must have passed this way, _______ there is no other road.
19. _______ respected, he is not liked.
20. _______ you are not ready we must go on.

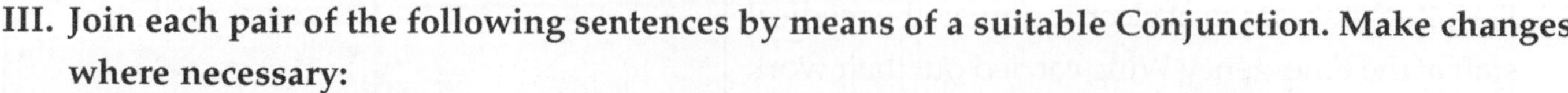

**III. Join each pair of the following sentences by means of a suitable Conjunction. Make changes where necessary:**

1. My sister is well. My brother is ill.
2. He sells carrots. He sells tomatoes.
3. She did not reach the goal. She worked hard.

4. They were poor. They were honest.
5. We love Browny. He is a faithful dog.
6. The musicians played. The students danced.
7. Rustom works hard. Ahmed is idle.
8. He is slow. He is sure.
9. I know. She does not think so.
10. You are tall. My sister is taller.
11. I will bring your dress. You wish it.
12. She tried to get up. She could not.
13. We went early to the theater. We could not get a seat.
14. Staff nurse Jeeth does not write fast. He writes well.
15. You must be tired. You have walked twelve miles.
16. The soldiers remained cheerful. They have been wounded.
17. She came. She was unwilling.
18. Ruksana lost the first rank. She tried her best.
19. The boy is here. The girl is here.
20. Doctors are respected. Doctors cure diseases.

So, to help you recall all about conunctions, here is a chart.

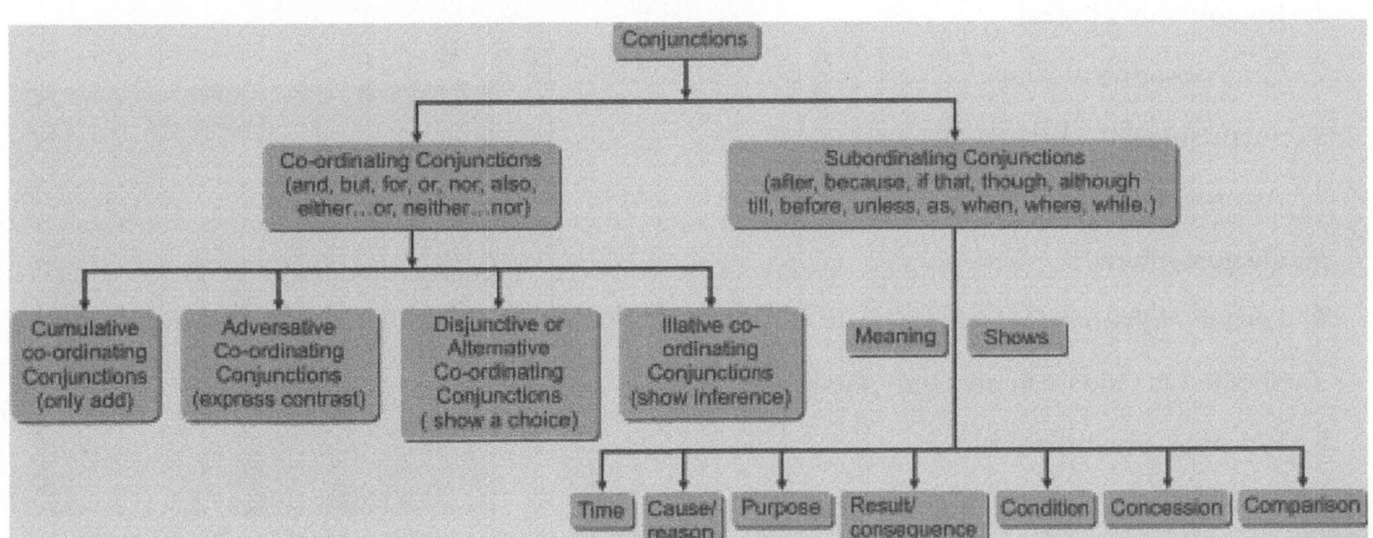

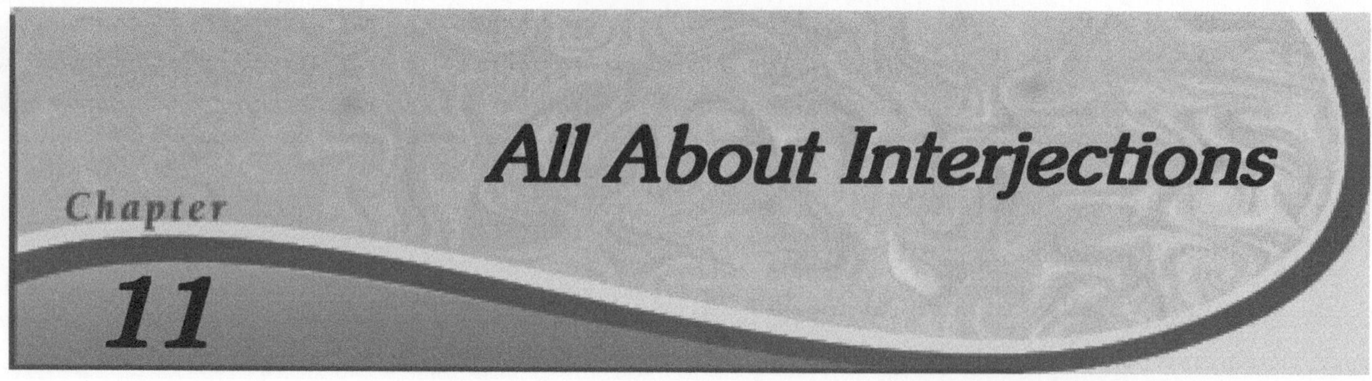

# Chapter 11 All About Interjections

Look at these sentences:

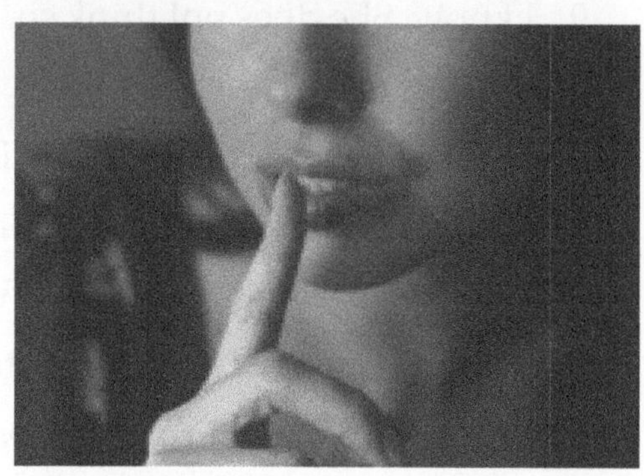

1. Aaha! Caught you eating chocolates.
2. Oh my God! I'll lose my job.
3. Hello! What are you doing here?
4. Oh! This corridor stinks!
5. Hush! Be silent.

The above sentences express disapproval, dismay, surprise, disgust, and warning.

This is shown by words **Aaha! Oh my God! Hello! Oh! Hush!**

***Definition:*** Words which express some sudden emotion or feeling are called as **interjections.**

The exclamatory mark (!) shows emotions or feelings.

Interjections may express:

1. Joy- hurrah! Huzza!
2. Grief or sadness- Alas!
3. Surprise- Hello! What! Oh! Gosh!
4. Approval- Well done!
5. Disgust- Phew!
6. Dismay- Oh boy!
7. Shock- Oh God! , Oh my God! , Gosh!
8. Warning- Hush! Sshhh!
9. Disapproval- Aaha! , For shame!

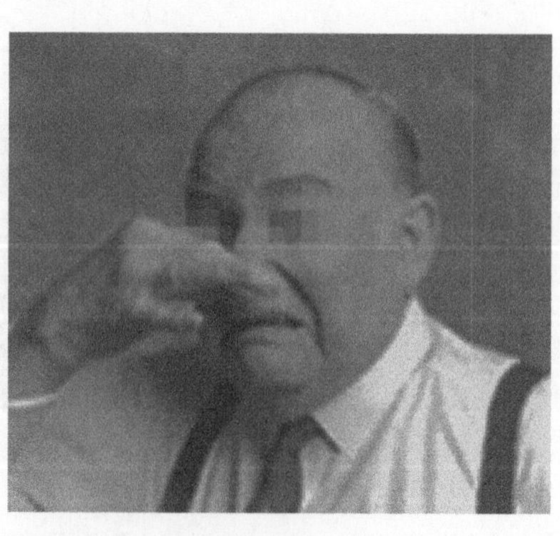

10. Admiration- Crikey!, Gee!, Cumbs!
11. Regret- What a pity! Oh! No! Ah me!
12. Anger- What a nuisance! For goodness sake!

## Exercises

**I. Express the emotion in each sentence:**

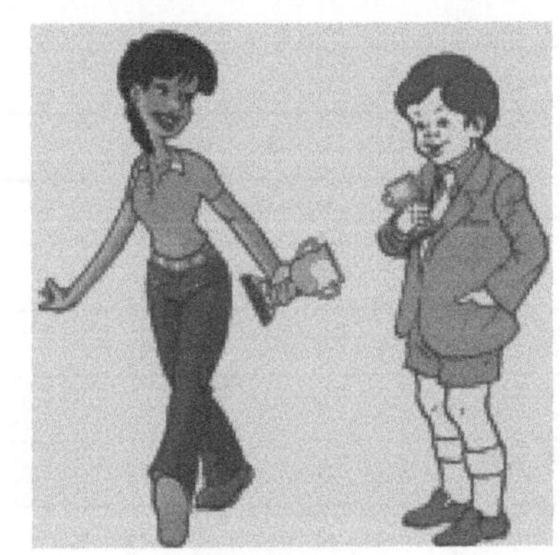

1. Oh! What a beautiful girl! ____________
2. What a man! Can't believe he is 70 years. ____________
3. Oh my God! I can't get up! ____________
4. Hurrah! We won all the prizes. ____________
5. Well done! The diagnosis is perfect. ____________
6. Gee! You fought well! ____________
7. Hush! The babies are sleeping. ____________
8. Alas! The child died in the night! ____________
9. Oh boy! I forgot to study the nursing reports again. ____________
10. For shame! All the reports have to be redone. ____________
11. Hello! Where are you going? ____________
12. Gosh! He is in ICU! ____________
13. What! Are you out of your mind? ____________
14. For goodness sake! Stop shouting. ____________
15. Phew! The patient's leg is so smelly! ____________

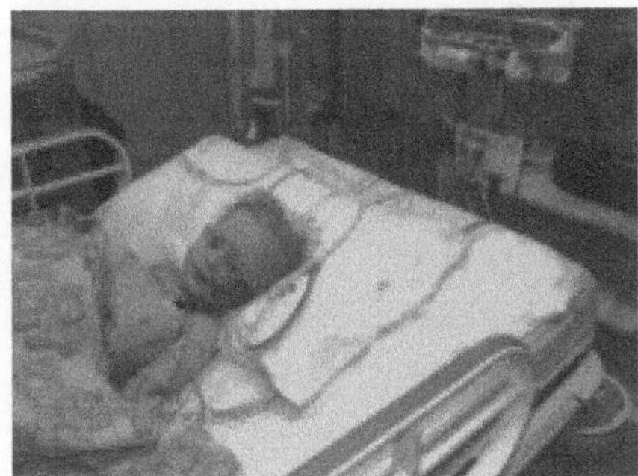

**II. Using any five interjections write a small paragraph describing emotions you underwent this week while on duty.**

______________________________________________________________________

______________________________________________________________________

______________________________________________________________________

______________________________________________________________________

______________________________________________________________________

______________________________________________________________________

______________________________________________________________________

______________________________________________________________________

______________________________________________________________________

______________________________________________________________________

______________________________________________________________________

______________________________________________________________________

______________________________________________________________________

______________________________________________________________________

______________________________________________________________________

______________________________________________________________________



With this, we come to the end of parts of speech. With constant practice you can master your English. Remember, any beginner will make mistakes. Just as a small child learns to walk, you have to keep trying to do exercises. Give a smile and pat yourself standing in front of the mirror every time you master a Chapter in this part. Watch how your confidence increases every time you do this.

Stay with me for the next interesting part.

Bye for now.

# Chapter 12: Question Forms

Wherever we go, we are curious to know about something. It can be about the place or food or people around us or events that have taken place - literally anything that catches our fancy. To get information, we ask different kinds of questions. We ask questions in different ways.

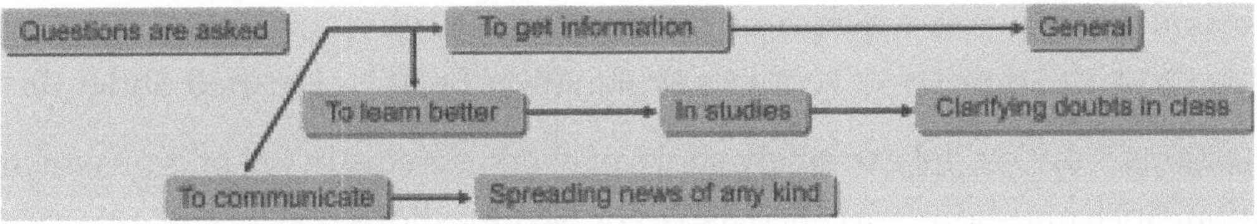


This brings us to the questions themselves. Look at these:

1. When do we have to submit the assignment?
2. How is the little girl in bed 4?
3. Are the band aids available in your shop?
4. Do you have the Child Development textbook?
5. Where do you live?
6. You saw the accident happen, didn't you?
7. Did the old man take his medicines?
8. Jenny is taller than Radha. Isn't she?
9. Which train reaches Delhi on Tuesday?
10. Does Shatabdi Express go to Delhi from Bangaluru?

Questions 1, 2, 5, 9 and 10 ask questions for which the answer should be given depending on the question asked and the situation. The answers usually are given in complete sentences. Now look at questions 3, 4, 7. Just saying yes or no will give the answer. Thus, they become one word answers.

Questions 6 and 7 show that the question is asked to emphasize a certain point.

Thus, we can say there are 3 types of questions:

1. Wh questions
2. Yes/No questions and
3. Question tags or Tag questions

So, we see in the questions, 1 to 10, that, 1,2,5,9 and 10 ask for information which requires some explanations (long answers). Such questions are called as 'Wh questions'. They are questions that start with the question words, what, where, which, when, whose ,why, how. Only 'How' stands out in this, but, the answer to a question 'how?' requires explanation. So, it is classified under this.

In the questions 3, 4, 7 we get extremely short answers, especially yes or no—which does not allow for explanation. Such questions are called as Yes or No Questions.

In the questions 6 and 8 there is no straight forward questioning as shown above. The question words are like tags (price tags attached to clothing) attached to a statement for confirmation or for support from others. Such question words are called as Question Tags.

Now there are many instances when questions are asked and they do not fall under the above three categories. Like these,

be (form) verbs, auxiliary verbs, verbs in simple present tense and verbs in simple past tense.

***Examples:***

Be- form verbs: am, is, are, was, and were. (been, being, be) When these verbs are used, they are always placed at the beginning of the question.

1. The children are all homesick. Are the children homesick?
2. This is a boarding school for international students. Is this an international boarding school?
3. The flood was the cause of waterborne infections. Was the waterborne infections caused by the flood?
4. All of us were immunized by Dr Suresh. Were all of us immunized by Dr Suresh?

# Question Forms

***Example:***

Auxiliary verbs: can, could have, has, had, must, shall should, will, would

1. I *could* breathe properly after I took dimox.

   Could I breathe properly after I took dimox?

2. The trekker *will* reach the base-camp shortly.

   Will the trekker reach the base-camp soon?

3. The rock climber *has* fallen down.

   Has the rock climber fallen down?

4. They *have* missed the details in histology lab.

   Have they missed the details in histology lab class?

5. The children had gone to bed hungry.

   Had the children gone to bed hungry?

6. The operation must be performed.

   Must the operation be performed?

7. New mothers shall not be allowed to lift weights.

   Shall the new mothers be allowed to lift weights?

8. In cold weather you should not get wet.

   Should you get wet in cold weather?

9. They would all leave together early.

   Would they all leave together early?

> ***Note:*** For questions formed by be- form verbs and auxiliary verbs, the answer can be in the Yes or No format.

*Example:* **Let us take the earlier examples.**

Has the rock climber fallen down?

No, he/she has not.

Or

Yes, he/she has.

Are the children homesick?

Yes, they are.

Or

No, they are not.



## Exercises

**I. Change the following sentences into, 'Yes/No' questions:**

1. The scalpel is used.

 ______________________________

2. Rudra is admitted to the hospital.

 ______________________________

3. Her arm was removed from the sling an hour ago.

 ______________________________

4. Head nurse Lavanya is strict.

 ______________________________

5. Head nurse Lavanya is neat.

 ______________________________

6. Cosmetics are expensive.

 ______________________________

7. This corridor leads to Radiology department.

 ______________________________

8. Skin has several layers.

9. Nurse Shanti is in ward 17.

10. The red-light in traffic lights means a stop signal.

**II. Change the following sentences containing auxiliary verbs into questions:**

1. Rita can walk for 15 minutes after the surgery.

2. Mohammed Saad could have inherited hypertension from his father.

3. Doctors have the power to heal.

4. The old man has gangrene.

5. Ella must learn to discipline her son.

6. I shall be honest with myself first.

7. The people should practice good manners.

8. My grandmother had the ability to remember people and their names.

9. Baby Dhruva will sleep well.

10. Nurse Shanta would bring the food tray everyday to my grand-father.

**III. Change these sentences with be-form verbs into questions:**

1. I am immunized against small pox.

   ______________________________

2. The doctor is ill today.

   ______________________________

3. They are the victims of plague.

   ______________________________

4. A patient with Chikun-gunya was treated today.

   ______________________________

5. All were feeling depressed.

   ______________________________



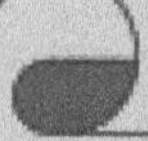

*Now let us consider the sentences which have the Verbs in the simple present tense.*

*The questions begin with Do/Does in this case.*

*'Do' is used when the subject is plural and 'Does' is used when the subject is in singular.*

***Like:***

*He looks rested today.*

*Does he look rested today?*

*The girls giggle in the class.*

*Do the girls giggle in class?*

***Remember:** When 'Does' is used the verb form changes.*

**IV. Change these sentences into questions:**

1. WBC builds up the immunity in the body.

______________________________

2. We often go out for long walks in the evening.

______________________________

3. A doctor ensures the confidences of their patients.

______________________________

4. Rajini applies moisturizer to her skin when she has a wash.

______________________________

5. Ramps help the physically handicapped to make their way into the mall.

______________________________

6. She monitors the children closely.

______________________________

7. They do not follow instructions carefully.

______________________________

8. The sun rises in the east.

______________________________

9. They meet us everyday.

______________________________

10. Mohan brings the post on Saturdays.

______________________________

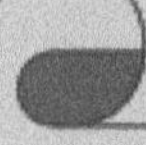

*Now look at these sentences which have the verb in the simple past tense. Such sentences change into questions with the word 'Did'.*

***Like:***

*The doctor gave me an injection to reduce the pain quickly.*

*Did the doctor give me an injection to reduce the pain quickly?*

*Deepak lost all his blood in the accident that killed him.*

*Did Deepak lose all his blood in the accident that killed him?*

***Remember:*** *The Verb form changes (gave to give) when 'Did' is used to form the question.*

**V. Frame questions using 'Did':**

1. The maid poured some cleaning solution into the water before cleaning the floor.

   ______________________________

2. They bought a new incubator.

   ______________________________

3. We girls went to see a late-night movie.

   ______________________________

4. TATA steel was established by Nasarwanji Tata.

   ______________________________

5. I took a painkiller to ease the pain in my legs.

   ______________________________

6. Jasmine drank soluble aspirin to ease the joint pain.

_______________________________________________

7. You went out last night.

_______________________________________________

8. Mr Brown died ten years ago.

_______________________________________________

9. The maid broke the expensive dish.

_______________________________________________

10. The children drank the milk and ate some biscuits.

_______________________________________________



**VI. Passage 1: Allergy to Penicillin**

Very high levels of penicillin can be tolerated by man. There are, however, number cases of allergic or hypersensitive reactions leading to death. According to recent concepts this sensitivity is caused by certain derivatives of penicillin associated with the pure molecule of penicillin. A skin test done with the penicillin to be injected to see hypersensitive reaction, if any, is a useful safeguard against such unfortunate fatalities.

**Based on the above passage give Yes/No answers to the questions given below:**

1. Can man tolerate high levels of pencillin?

_______________________________________________

2. There are no allergic cases known when penicillin is adminstered. Comment.

_______________________________________________

3. Is a skin test needed before injecting penicillin?

_______________________________________________

4. The concept of sensitivity to penicillin, is it recent?

_______________________________________________

5. Did the treatment of patients change in hospital after the discovery of sulphanilamides, penicillin and streptomycin?

_______________________________________________

6. Did the discovery of new medicine promise that diseases might be brought under control?

_______________________________________________

7. Will infections respond dramatically to chemotherapy?

_______________________________________________

8. In spite of antibiotics do the staphylococcal infection persist?

_______________________________________________



**VII. Passage 2: Antibiotics**

The younger generation of people born the post World War II era (after 1945) may not quite realize the magnitude of the problem faced by doctors when treating their parents and grandparents for infectious diseases before the advent of antibiotics. Today, thanks to the outstanding scientific contribution of the older generation, it is taken for granted that most disease-producing microbes can be eradicated by one drug or another. Before 1945, medical wards in hospitals always had a large number of young people seriously ill with diseases such as pneumonia, meningitis, septicaemia, while the post-operation wards were filled with patients having pus oozing out of abscesses, carbuncles and improper healing of surgical wounds. Now all this is changed due to the discovery of sulphanilamides, penicillin, streptomycin and a large array of antibiotics discovered in recent years. The advent of sulphanilamide drugs and antibiotics brought with it the promise that bacterial diseases might be brought under control, but that promise has not been fulfilled. Although many infections respond dramatically to chemotheraphy, tuberculosis, dysentery and typhoid fever continue to be endemic in many parts of the world, while cholera and plague erupt periodically; staphylococcal infection persists in the most advanced hospitals. One major reason for this is that the microorganisms have developed resistance to drugs.

When penicillin came on the scene it could easily eradicate staphylococci. However, by the mid-1950's as many as 90 percent of staphylococcal infections seen in hospital wards were associated with penicillin-resistant strains. Cholramphenicol and erythromycin were fortunately discovered in time to deal with the penicillin-resistant staphylococci and now, where strains resistant to all the three antibiotics are appearing, other synthetic derivatives of penicillin have been produced to deal with them.

**Based on the given passage give `Yes/No' answers to the questions given below:**

1. Do the younger generation of people born in the post-World War II era reallize the magnitude of the problems faced by doctors?

   ______________________________________________

2. Were these problems due to the non-availability of antibiotics?

   ______________________________________________

3. Has the older generation contributed a lot in scientific research?

   ______________________________________________

4. Did the medical wards in 1945 house a large number of seriously young people?

   ______________________________________________

**VIII. Passage 3**

**After reading the passage, construct 5 `Yes/No' questions and 5 `Do' or `Did' questions:**

Khangchendzonga is the world's third highest mountain peak. It is in Sikkim in north-east part of India. It is considered as the toughest mountain to summit (climb and stand on the top of the peak). In spite of extreme dangers, climbers from all over the world attempt it. Here is a small incidence of one such attempt.

Mountaineering equipment and skills have developed much since Khangchendzonga was first attempted in 1905, but no technology, no condition can prepare a person to remain stuck in their tents for 36 hours at a stretch at 7,400 metres while storm rages outsides. German climber Ralf Diymovits and Austrian Gerlinde Kalfenbrunner were similarly grounded while attempting the mountain in April-May 2005 on the fiftieth anniversary of the first ascent with temperature plunging to twenty degrees celsius below zero inside the tent, the storm was forcing snow inside the tent through the breathing slits, humidity was high and the high velocity winds outside collided with the synthetic fibres of their tents to spark off miniature lightning displays zigzagging across the tents. To spend 36 excruciating hours getting battered by snow and ice and knowing all along that the eventual push to the summit, if it was at all allowed by the weather, would demand hands-on rock climbing is a disturbing thought that can disorient the most seasoned of climbers. That is what Khangchendzonga is all about, a mind-numbing assortment of contrasting challenges. Ice falls, ice melts, soft snow, avalanches and howling winds hound climbers from base camp to the summit, the approach to which requires walking and even climbing on exposed rock!

1.

2.

3.

4.

5.

6.

7.

8.

9.

10.



**IX. Passage 4**

**After reading the passage, construct 5 `Yes/No' questions and 5 `Do' or `Did' questions:**

Dew and frost both occur on still clear nights. Heavy dews usually follow warm days during which a great deal of water is evaporated into the air from streams, lakes and puddles. When the sun set, the ground cools rapidly if there is no cloud, and so does the layer of air close to it. Some of the water vapour in this layer condenses and forms dew.

When the ground and the layer of air close to it cool below freezing point, the water vapour condenses as ice crystals, or frost. Fog is thick mist and is formed in just the same way. At sea, mist or fog is caused by warm air blowing over the cooler water of the sea.

1.

2.

3.

4.

5.

6.

7.________________________________________

8.________________________________________

9.________________________________________

10._______________________________________

**Let us now study the three types of questions.**

## WH Questions

These are 7 kinds (Wh-questions). These are helpful in getting explanation and details about a person, situation, event, object or place. There are 6 Wh questions and 1 question starting with H. Together they are called as Wh questions.

These are why, what, when, where, who, which and how.

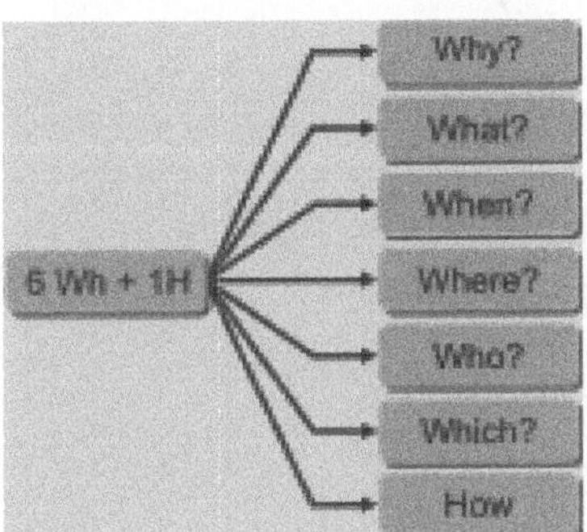


**Let us now acquaint ourselves with their usage.**

*Why:* This is used to know the reason or the cause of an event.

*What:* This is used to know more about an object, activity, opinion, etc.

*When:* This is used to know more about the time or date of an event or incident.

*Where:* This is used to know more about a place, an event, situation or activity.

*Who:* This is used to know more about a person or a group of people only.

*Which:* This is used to know more about particular details. This is also used more to elicit descriptive explanations to help further understanding of events.

*How:* This is used to know more about the condition of an event, activity or happening.

*Whose, whom* - used to show possession and particulars.

***Examples:***

1. Why did they close the college?

   They closed as there was no infrastructure.
2. Why did her hands shake as she signed the hospital papers?

   The enormity of the responsibilities she was shouldering made her hands shake as she signed the hospital papers.
3. Why can't we go on a picnic today?

   We can't go on a picnic today because it is cloudy.
4. What is the seminar about?

   The seminar is about AIDS.
5. What is your father's occupation?

   My father is a doctor.
6. What will happen to the children now?

   The parents died in the accident. The children survived.
7. When will I be appointed as a class teacher?

   You will be appointed as a class teacher soon.
8. When did you suffer from Rheumatic fever?

   I suffered from Rheumatic fever when I was a teenager.
9. When did the dentist examine his jaw?

   The dentist examined his jaw this morning.
10. Where did I get my physiotherapy done?

    I got my physiotherapy done at MSA hospital.
11. Where is the first-aid kit in this van?

    The first-aid kit is kept near the driver in this van.
12. Where is the rock-show taking place?

    The rock-show is at the Wong stadium.

13. Who told you to clean the windows?

    Arti told me to clean the windows.

14. Who gave you the medicine?

    Nurse Elize gave me the medicine.

15. Who cheated in the examination?

    Rajiv cheated in the examination.

16. Which arm is hurt?

    The right arm is hurt (not what arm is hurt)

17. Which room on this floor belongs to sister Lea?

    The third room along the corridor belongs to sister Lea.

18. Which red blouse is yours?

    The blouse with the lightest shade of red is mine.

19. How did she get her fingers disfigured?

    She got her fingers disfigured in the fire.

20. How does Dr Kiran listen to his child patients?

    Dr Kiran listens attentively.

21. How is the new pathologist in his work?

    The new pathologist is very meticulous in his work.

**X. Choose the correct form of Wh- questions given in the box and fill in the blanks:**

| Why, what, when, where, who, which, how whose, whom |
|---|

1. _________ is there? _________ are you?
2. _________ is the matter with Dr Rao? He is angry.
3. She asked, "_________ cup would you like the best?"

4. __________ is this dissection box?
5. __________ did you see?
6. __________ did Abdul go yesterday?
7. ___________ many boys are in your team?
8. This is the reason _________ she left hurriedly.
9. _________ will the lecture session begin?
10. _________ comes first? The egg or the chicken?
11. __________ will the CAT scan be performed?
12. __________ do you feel after the operation?
13. _________ are the nurses worried?
14. _________ did you consult with your case?
15. _________ help will you take once you go home?



**XI. Some sentences are given below. Let's see if you can frame Wh-questions that suit the sentences. To help you, the key words are highlighted:**

1. This football is **Sanjeev's**.

   ______________________________________________

2. You can trust **Anna Hazare** in this matter.

   ______________________________________________

3. **Sheetal** is studying nursing.

   ______________________________________________

4. My friend Sandhya gave birth to her son at **6 am**.

   ______________________________________________

5. The house surgeons relax in the **Duty Doctor's room.**

   ______________________________________________

6. Dr.Ratna **felt sad** on seeing the terminally ill child in bed 9.

______________________________________________

7. **Florence Nightingale Award** was given to Nagaratna today.

______________________________________________

8. **I went to the movie** yesterday.

______________________________________________

9. They **felt fine** after seeing a doctor.

______________________________________________

10. Alekhya came here **yesterday**.

______________________________________________



**XII. Frame Wh-questions after reading the Passage below:**

## Whither Antibiotic Therapy?

The younger generation of people born the post world war II era (after 1945) may not quite realize the magnitude of the problem faced by doctors when treating their parents and grandparents for infectious diseases before the advent of antibiotics. Today, thanks to the outstanding scientific contribution of the older generation, it is taken for granted that most disease-producing microbes can be eradicated by one drug or another. Before 1945, medical wards in hospitals always had a large number of young people seriously ill with diseases such as pneumonia, meningitis, septicaemia, while the post-operation wards were filled with patients having pus oozing out of abscesses, carbuncles and improper healing of surgical wounds. Now all this is changed due to the discovery of sulphanilamides, penicillin, streptomycin and a large array of antibiotics discovered in recent years. The advent of sulphanilamide drugs and antibiotics brought with it the promise that bacterial diseases might be brought under control, but that promise has not been fulfilled. Although many infections respond dramatically to chemotherapy, tuberculosis, dysentery and typhoid fever continue to be endemic in many parts of the world, while cholera and plague erupt periodically; staphylococcal infection persists in the most advanced hospitals. One major reason for this is that the microorganisms have developed resistance to drugs.

When penicillin came on the scene it could easily eradicate staphylococci. However, by the mid-1950's as many as 90 per cent of staphylococcal infections seen in hospital wards were associated with penicillin-resistant strains. Cholramphenicol and erythromycin were fortunately discovered in time to deal with the penicillin-resistant staphylococci and now, where strains resistant to all the three antibiotics are appearing, other synthetic derivatives of penicillin have been produced to deal with them.

1. ______________________________

2. ______________________________

3. ______________________________

4. ______________________________

5. ______________________________

6. ______________________________

7. ______________________________

8. ______________________________

9. ______________________________

10. ______________________________



**XIII. Here is a fun activity to know if you have understood the Wh-question format. Frame as many Wh-questions based on the three sentences given below:**

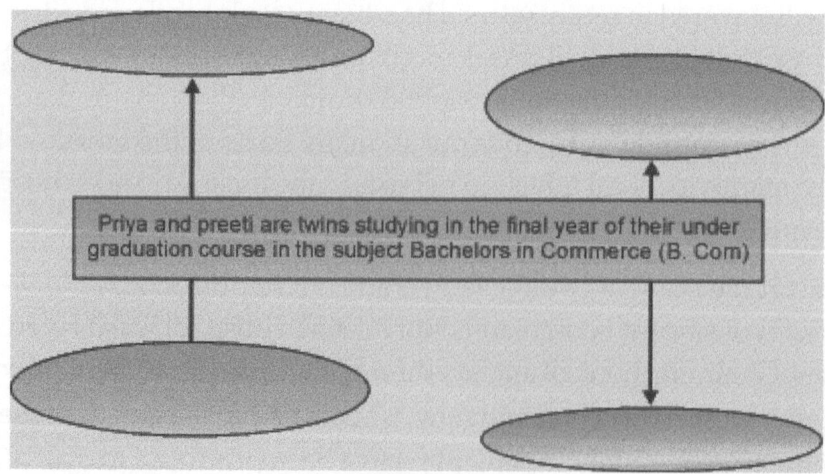

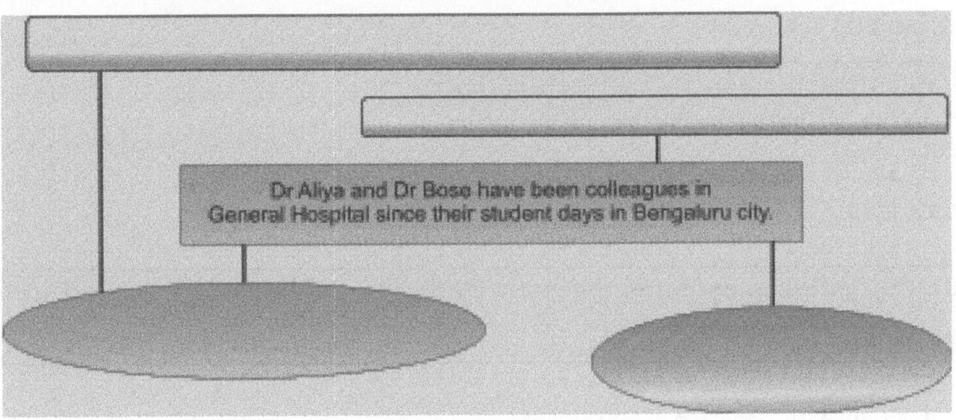


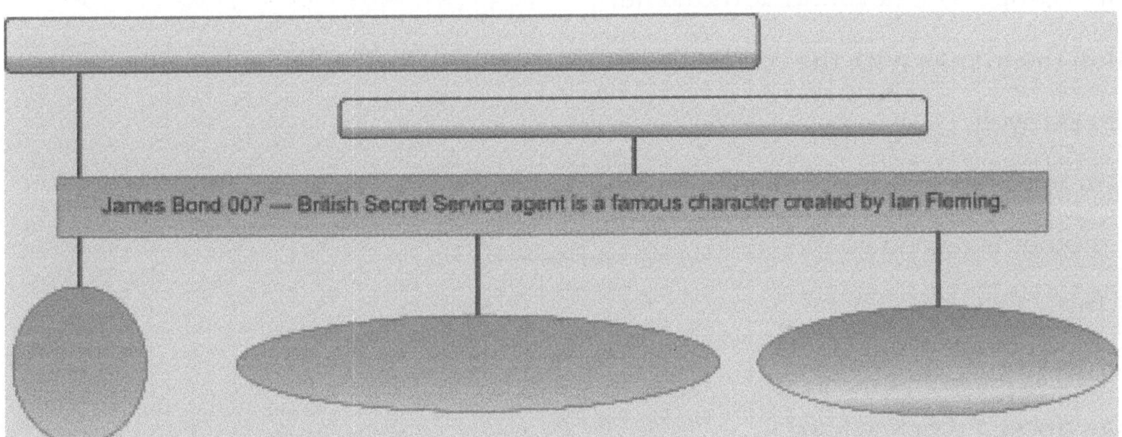




So, now you can see for yourself how a single statement can have multiple questions. Reminds you of children asking a lot of questions without getting tired, right?

Lets move on to the next question form.

## Question Tags

You would have noticed while having conversations, a statement is made and a confirmation is asked in the same breath. Like : "It's very cold, isn't it?"

The question part is called a question tag.

> ***Note:*** If the statement is positive, the Question Tag is Negative.

Auxiliary + n't + subject

*Example:* It's raining, isn't it?

If the statement is negative, the question tag is positive.

Auxiliary + subject

*Example:* He isn't busy, is he?

*Note:* When the sentence contains the main verb, the auxiliary 'do' is used in the question tag.

She appears complacent, doesn't she?

He lost his fingers in the foundry, didn't he?

**XIV. Fill in the blanks with the correct Question-tags:**

1. He can ski well, ______________?
2. William broke the garden frame, ________________?
3. Your mother is a good cook, __________________?
4. He is free, __________?
5. He can't skate, _____________?
6. Raghav doesn't practice hard, _____________?
7. The children haven't arrived yet, ________________?
8. It's very depressing today, _____________?
9. You love her, ____________?
10. Dr Naina will come, ____________?
11. Your parents are doctors, ___________________?
12. They have sold the library, ______________?
13. She needn't get up early today, ________________?
14. It isn't ready yet, _______________?
15. Mr Pandey is diagnosed with Parkinson's disease, ______________?

16. Smelly underarms are an embarrassment, __________?

17. Children must have eight hours' sleep, ______________?

18. The child is unable to respond to colour stimulus, ____________?

19. The nurses prepared all the surgical equipments needed in the surgery, __________?

20. The patient looks healthy, _____________?

21. Walking as an exercise prevents many ailments, ______________?

22. The briefing started at 8:30, _____________?

23. She looks lost, ________________?

24. High Altitude Sickness leads to pulmonary edema, __________?

25. Lots of fluids should be ingested to prevent dehydration, ________________?

**XV. Choose the correct answer:**

1. _________________ does one turn to when all doors close?

   (a) Who (c) Which

   (b) Whom (d) God

2. There is a significant link between breathlessness and High Altitude Sickness, __________?

   (a) isn't it? (c) ain't it?

   (b) why (d) don't it?

3. The best age to become a mother is in one's twenties, _____________?

   (a) which is? (c) doesn't it?

   (b) isn't it? (d) none of the above.

4. The injection didn't pain, ________________?

   (a) didn't it? (c) did it?

   (b) does it? (d) do it?

5. Public Health Care System must be better managed, _____________?

   (a) mustn't it? (c) might it?

   (b) must it not? (d) shouldn't it?

6. ____________ gave the flower to Aliya?

   (a) Whom (c) Which

   (b) Who (d) What

7. ____________ the doctors know the change in rules this week?

   (a) Does (c) Which

   (b) Do (d) What

8. _____________ do I keep these washed clothes?

   (a) When (c) Do

   (b) Where (d) Will

9. Software engineers are known to have erratic eating habits, __________?

   (a) aren't they? (c) won't they?

   (b) will they? (d) how

10. BPO employees have disturbed sleeping patterns, __________?

    (a) don't they (c) do they

    (b) haven't they (d) why won't they

With this you have reached a comfortable level in your English. If you have doubts, go back, check and clarify them. From the first chapter till here, you have covered all aspects of grammar that one should know to hold a reasonably good conversation in English. You will be able to understand much more than you did earlier.

Remember to listen to Radio, watch News on TV, sing songs (in tune or out-of-tune don't bother) in English and read English Newspapers and magazines. In no time at all, you will be able to do more in English than you ever thought that you could.

# Part II

- Transformation of Sentences
- Direct and Indirect Speech

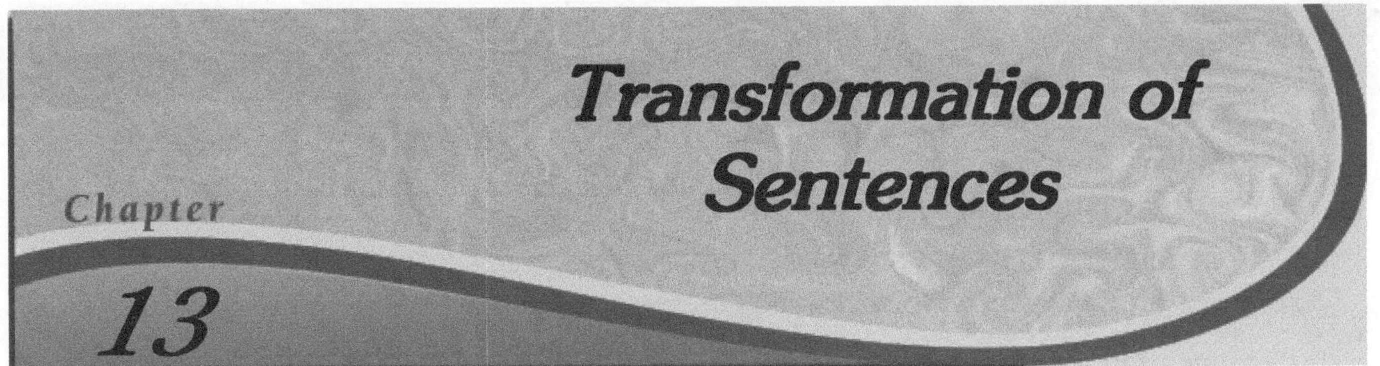


# Chapter 13: Transformation of Sentences

In Chapter 2, we got to know that any sentence is divided into two parts–Subject and Predicate along with four different types of sentences.

Then we got to know about phrase and clause. Now we continue with the next aspect of sentences.

Sentences can be further divided into three types. They are:

1. Simple Sentences
2. Compound Sentences, and
3. Complex Sentences.

**What are these sentences ? We shall know all about them.**

**Look at these Sentences:**

1. Dr Ajay's diagnosis cured his illness.
2. This book is mine.
3. The nurses have boarded the bus.
4. She might come home today.

All the four Sentences have one subject, one predicate and one verb.

1. Dr Ajay's—diagnosis | cured | his illness

| Subject | Verb | Predicate |
|---|---|---|
| Dr Ajay's—diagnosis | cured | his illness |

2. This book | is | mine

| Subject | Verb | Predicate |
|---|---|---|
| This book | is | mine |

Now you identify the subject, verb, predicate for the next two sentences.

3. ________________________________________

4. ________________________________________

Before we begin, let us spend some time on the clause.

In Chapter 2, Phrase and Clause have been explained so we move on to the next aspect of 'Clause'. Clauses can be divided into two kinds:

Independent or principal or Main clause

and

Dependent/ or subordinate clause

Look at this sentence:

If you don't fix the tap, it will continue to drip.

*Note:*

(Here drip water is wrong. Water is understood. So it need not be written)



It is made up of two parts:

i. If you don't (do not) fix the *tap*
ii. The tap will continue to drip

Each part contains a subject and predicate of its own, for example

i. *If you* — Subject; *don't fix the tap* — Predicate

ii. *It* — Subject; *will continue to drip* — Predicate

Therefore each part is called a Clause.

*If* is the conjunction which joins the two sentences into one. We also notice that both the sentences make good sense by themselves, and can stand all by themselves as a complete sentence. So, each clause is *independent* of the other. It can be of the same order or rank.

Thus it is called a Principal or Main clause or an Independent clause.

**A sentence can have more than one main clause.**

# Transformation of Sentences

A sentence which has only *one* subject and *one* predicate is called as a Simple Sentence.

Now see these sentences:

1. The moon rose and every thing looked silvery.
2. The torch was bright so we could see our way.
3. We were caught in a political rally but we still made it on time.
4. The vaccine might work or it might not work.

You will notice that:

Each sentence is made up of two simple sentences

They are joined by conjunctions like 'and' , 'but', 'or', 'so', for

Let us see how this is possible.

1. The moon rose (simple sentence)
2. Everything looked silvery (simple sentence)

When these two simple sentences are put together, we get

1. The moon rose *and* everything looked silvery.

   These two parts are joined by the conjunction *and*

2. The torch was bright (simple sentence)
3. We could see our way (simple sentence)

Putting the two sentences at together, we get

The torch war bright *so* we could see our way.

Each part contains a subject and a predicate of its own.

| Like | *The moon* | *rose* |
|---|---|---|
| | Sub | Predicate and verb |
| | *Everything* | *looked silvery* |
| | Sub | Verb Predicate |

Therefore each part is a sentence which in turn is part of a larger sentence. In other words each part is a clause and is independent of each other. So such a sentence is called as a compound sentence .

A sentence, which is made up of two or more clauses, is called a Compound Sentence. Now see this sentence.

Now look at this sentence

They sang when night came.

The two parts of the sentence are:

i. They sang

ii. When night came

Each part contains a subject and a predicate of its own and forms part of a large sentence. Each part is a clause.

| | | |
|---|---|---|
| i. *They* | *Sang* | |
| Sub | Predicate | |
| ii. When | *night* | *came* |
| | Sub | Predicate |



We also notice something else. The clause *They sang*, makes good sense all by itself. Hence, it can stand all by itself. Therefore it is called the Principal clause or the Main Clause.

The clause *when night came* makes sense, but not complete sense. Hence, it cannot stand all by itself as a complete sentence. It depends on *they sang*. Therefore, it is called the Dependent or Subordinate Clause.

In this sentence, *They sang when night came*, has main clause and one subordinate clause.

In the sentence, *If you don't fix the tap, it will continue to drip*, there are two main clauses. Thus a conjunction 'if' is joining the two sections of the sentence.

The first sentence is a complex sentence and the second sentence is compound sentence as two simple sentences join with the conjunction *if*.

That is

If you don't fix tap both the clauses are independent by themselves and make perfect sense

conjunction

It (tap) will continue to drip

Now let us know more about these two sentences.

Night came on and rain fell heavily and the ambulance crew got wet.

Here we gave 3 simple sentences each consists of three main clauses.

i. Night came on

ii. Rain fell heavily

iii. The ambulance crew got wet

This kind of a sentence is also called a compound sentence.

Therefore the earlier definition of a compound sentence can be modified like this

A Compound sentence is one made up two or more main clauses.

> ***Note:*** Some Grammar books also use the term 'Double' here for these kinds of sentences 'Multiple' is used for a sentence of *more than two* main clauses.

Next observe these sentences:

1. Nurse Sharon rested when evening came
2. As the students entered the room, the teacher said she would not allow them to sit.
3. The trekkers started their trek as day broke.

Sentences 1 and 3 consist of two parts:

1. i. Nurse Sharon rested

   ii. When evening came

3 iii. The trekkers started their trek

   iv. As day broke

Each part contains a subject and a predicate of its own and forms part of a large sentence, therefore, each part is a clause.

We observe that Nurse Sharon rested and the trekkers started their trek make good sense all by themselves. Thus, they can stand by themselves as a complete sentence. Therefore it is called the **Main or Principal clause.**

The clause (ii) when evening came and (iv) as day broke cannot stand by themselves and make good sense. They are dependent on their Principal or Main clauses. They are thus called as **Dependent or Subordinate clause.**

In sentence 2, there are three clauses:

i. The teacher said (Main clause)

ii. As the students entered the room (Subordinate clause)

iii. She would not allow them to sit (Subordinate clause).

Such a sentence is also called as a complex sentence,

Thus, a sentence which consists of one main clause and one or more subordinate clauses is said to be a **Complex sentence.**



## Exercises

**I. Write 'I' for independent clause and 'D' for dependent clause.**

1. Nurse George went to the cafeteria
2. Since doctors went to the movie
3. Pluto was purring
4. Nurse Saritha and nurse Jasmine played chess
5. After Matorn Joan left for ER
6. While the table is being painted
7. If you have operated properly
8. Since I am in a hurry
9. Since nurse Manya has taken her exam in child psychology
10. Dr Bhatia nefused to talk to him

**II. Identify the simple, compound and complex sentences in the following:**

1. Walk quickly, else you will not overtake her.
2. The city in which I live is very large.

3. I called nurse Rasheeda, but she gave me no answer.
4. The management agreed to the architects' proposals, for they thought them reasonable.
5. They went because they were invited.
6. Nurse Gigi returned home because she was tired.
7. Any guest is unwelcome when he or she stays too long.
8. Man proposes, but good disposes.
9. God made the country and man made the town.
10. We must eat to live, but we should not live to eat.
11. The young mother who lost her infant must weep or she will go mad with grief.
12. The nurses had bread for breakfast.
13. The surgery is well lit.
14. The senior nurse hands the surgical instruments to the surgeon while the other nurses assist.
15. As the athelete fell on the tracks, the medical staff rushed from the tent with a stretcher and refused to allow him to walk.
16. Nurse Aiyna and nurse Babitha went to the labour ward after they had finished their coffee break.
17. The senior citizens had to wait inside the lounge as it was snowing
18. The book had not been lent for many years before I borrowed it
19. Although her friend has invited her to the wedding, she does not want to go.
20. I called the doctor's office several times but he was out

**III. Write the compound sentences given above in the space provided here and identify the clasuses and the conjunction.**

______________________________________________

______________________________________________

______________________________________________

______________________________________________

______________________________________________

**IV. Write the complex sentences you have identified in the above exercises here and identify the main clause and one or more subordinate clause in the space given below:**



## Conversion of Simple Sentences to Compound (Double) Sentences

We do not speak and write in our daily lives with clearly marked compound and complex sentences. Without our knowledge we would have used a simple sentence in a complex or compound sentence and vice-versa. Yes this means conversion of one kind of sentence into another possible. Let us see how to do this.

**I. Join the given pair of simple sentences to make compound sentences.**

Join the gives poir of simple sentences to make compound sentences.

1. I might study child psychology, tonight I might study clinics.

2. Nurse Radha likes novels. Nurse Stanley doesn't like novels.

3. The street was long. I was tired.

4. The scalpel was heavy. It was blunt.

___

5. The wheel chair is for patients. It is not for healthy people.

___

The above sentences are not what you would encounter in daily life. So how do you convert simple sentences to compound sentences in everyday life? Here is an example.

***Simple:*** She must work very hard to make up for the lost time.

***Compound:*** She must work very hard *and* make up for the lost time.

When we convert a simple sentence into a compound sentence, we have to add a word or a phrase into the clause. In the above sentence it is 'and'.

Look at this one.

***Simple:*** The baby has high fever, it also has diarrhoea.

***Compound:*** The baby not only has high fever but also diarrhoea.

Here *not only, but* have been added to convert the simple sentence into compound.

Now, convert the simple sentences given below into compound sentence.

1. In this room *sat the patient gazing* on the garden.

___

2. To everyone's *surprise, the experiment* completely failed.

___

3. Feeling a fever *coming on, I wore* warm clothes.

___

4. Being occupied *with important cases,* the surgeon had no leisure to see his friends.

___

5. Owing to floods *influenza* is everywhere.

______________________________________________

6. The doctors had not *completed* their work by sunset.

______________________________________________

7. *By her pleasant manners she gained many friends.*

______________________________________________

8. *On account of his negligence the child suffered from fever.*

______________________________________________

9. *Throwing off her uniform, she plunged into the swimming pool.*

______________________________________________

10. *Hearing the dietician's instructions the obese person walked away.*

______________________________________________



The question does arise, can we convert a compound sentence into a simple sentence? Yes, we can do it.

Look at these sentences.

***Compound:*** She finished her aerobic exercise and put away the mats.

***Simple:*** Having finished her aerobic exercises, she put away the mats.

***Compound:*** One must either pay the bill as soon as possible or endure water shortage.

***Simple:*** Failing prompt payment the water supply will be stopped.

***Compound:*** We must eat, or we cannot live.

***Simple:*** We must eat to live.

Now convert, the compound (Double) sentences given below into simple sentences.

1. They were sick, and often suffered great hardship

***Simple:***______________________________________________

2. Nurse Joy overslept himself, and so he missed the class.

***Simple:***________________________________________

3. This stethoscope cannot be mine, for it is too long.

***Simple:***________________________________________

4. This nurse worked hard, the management therefore made the nurse in-charge of the nursing station.

***Simple:***________________________________________

5. Her partner dies, and this added to her difficulties.

***Simple:***________________________________________

6. Make haste or else you will be late.

***Simple:***________________________________________

7. He is very intelligent, but he is humble.

***Simple:***________________________________________

8. My friend arrived and we talked for a long time.

***Simple:***________________________________________

9. I had no chocolates with me, and I could not give the child anything.

***Simple:***________________________________________

10. Be honest and you will be fearless

***Simple:***________________________________________



## Conversion of Simple Sentences into Complex Sentences

Observe these sentences:

1. ***(a) Simple:*** He confessed *to his crime.*

   ***(b) Complex:*** He confessed *that he was guilty.*

2. ***(a) Simple:*** Peter's *silence* proves his guilt.

   ***(b) Complex:*** *The fact that peter is silent* proves his guilt.

3. ***(a) Simple:*** Only officers are admitted.

   ***(b) Complex:*** *If you are not an officer* you cannot be admitted.

The second sentences (complex sentences) in each pair is got by expanding a word or phrase into subordinate clause.

For example: In sentence (1a) his crime is expanded in sentence (1b) to 'that he was guilty', guilty is the added word that has the meaning 'knowing that one has done wrong'.

In sentence (2a) silence an abstract noun is expanded to 'The fact that Peter is silent shows the reality that Peter is not talking.

Same way. In sentence (3) the complex sentence is formed by making the condition to enter the place very clear.

## Exercise

**Convert the following simple sentences to complex sentences:**

1. I expect to meet Dr Ali Khan today.

______________________________

2. The boys requested for the teacher's help.

______________________________

3. She is said to be billionaire.

______________________________

4. Tell the truth.

______________________________

5. Rita saw a wounded boy.

______________________________

6. The value of exercise is great.

______________________________

7. These are not the methods of research.

______________________________

8. She is an assistant nurse.

______________________________________________

9. Dr Bhat is feared for his anger

______________________________________________

10. The child would be quite happy with another toy now.

______________________________________________

11. That was done in his absence.

______________________________________________

12. Come back at 5 o'clock.

______________________________________________

13. There is no hope of their recovery.

______________________________________________

14. Inspite of her poor heath, she worked hard.

______________________________________________

15. Tell her your ideas.

______________________________________________

This will take us to the next step–conversion of complex sentences to simple sentences.

**Example:** *They said that they were innocent.*

This is a complex sentence.

*They declared their innocence.*

This becomes a simple sentence.

Which brings us back to the definition of simple and complex sentence when you apply the rule it becomes clear how the change occurred.

Ramu died in the village *where he was born.*

This is a complex sentence the words in italic show the clause.

Ramu died in his *native* village.

This gives facts in a simple way. Thus it is a simple sentence.

You may ask "Why should I know about this reverse conversion—complex to simple sentences? Haven't you come across people who talk in a long winding manner or read such sentences? At such times have not you wished that it was put across in a simple manner? Well, this shows how you can do such simplifications.

## Exercise



**Convert the following complex sentences into simple sentences:**

1. It is horrible that children should die of malnutrition.

   ______________________________

2. She was unable to hear what you were saying.

   ______________________________

3. If you turn to the left, you will reach the hospital.

   ______________________________

4. They went half-an-hour earlier, that they might get a good seat.

   ______________________________

5. The instructions are so complex that I cannot understand it.

   ______________________________

You will never realise that you've mastered this till you see somebody struggling to simplify instruction or making mistakes while taking in long sentences. Have a happy time as you go ahead and master this aspect of sentences.

We now move on to Direct and Indirect Speech.

Chapter 14

# Direct and Indirect Speech

We come to an interesting part of grammar. Everyday life and most of the grammar you have studied so far come in handy here. You must be wondering about what you read just now. Well, let me show you what I mean. First let us take all the grammar you have studied so far. Parts of speech, question forms, conversion of sentences have helped you in knowing and using English in a better way. You talk with many people in many situations in different ways everyday. You use all the grammar you have studied, in everyday life—talking and speaking. While talking or speaking, you do it in two ways. Either you talk or speak to whoever you want directly, or you tell someone all that was happening in front of you as the person was not present to witness all that has happened.

When you talk to people in exact words, it is called **Direct Speech.**

When you tell what was said by someone else without using the exact words, it is called ***Indirect*** or ***Reported Speech***.

***Example:*** Jenny said, "I am very tired now."
This is in Direct Speech.

Jenny said that she was very tired then.
This is in Indirect Speech.

We use more of reported speech in everyday life as it is difficult to remember the exact words of all that we hear and repeat them all exactly as we heard it to others. Direct speech is found more in the story books and in dramas.

What did you observe in the two sentences given above? If you haven't observed anything, do it now. Here is help for you to list your observations. If you still haven't observed, well, read this list and you will know what to obeserve in sentences. For those who have made the observations, you can confirm with the list below.

- The first sentence has double quotation marks (" ") and a comma (,).
- The second sentence does not have any.

This " " shows that a person is talking to another person. This mark shows the exact words of the speaker.

Now when the change from Direct Speech to Indirect Speech is done, like in the second sentence given above, certain changes will be noticed. They are:

- The conjunction 'that' is used before the Indirect statement. This use of 'that' does not take place while speaking English. It is only used during writing.
- Pronoun is changed.

  Here *I* is changed to *he.*
- Change of verb.

  Here *am* is changed to *was* (Present Tense is changed to Past Tense).
- Change of Adverb

  Here *now* is changed to *then.*

This brings us to the question "are there rules for changing Direct Speech into Indirect Speech?" The Answer is 'yes' there are certain basic rules one follows while changing one form of speech into another. They are given below.



### *Rule 1*

If the main verb is in the Present Tense in the Direct Speech, it is changed to the corresponding Past Tense in the Indirect Speech.

*Example:* **A.** A simple present tense becomes a simple past tense.

**Direct speech:** The patient said," I *am* tired".

**Indirect speech:** The patient said (that) he* *was* tired.

[*Here 'she' may also be used, as the gender is not specified]

**B.** A present continuous tense becomes a past continuous tense.

**Direct speech:** The nurse said, "Matron *is supervising* the junior nurses".

**Indirect speech:** The nurse said (that) matron *was supervising* the junior nurses.

**C.** A present perfect tense becomes a past perfect tense.

**Direct speech:** The teacher said, " *I have finished* the syllabus".

**Indirect speech:** The teacher said (that) he* had finished the syllabus.

[*Here 'she' may also be used, as the gender is not specified]

**Note:** *'Shall'* of the Future Tense is changed into *'should'*.
*'Will'* of the Future Tense is changed into *'would'* or *'should'*.

If in the Direct Speech, the simple past tense is used, it is changed to *past perfect* in the Indirect Speech.

*Example:* **Direct speech:** Namitha said, "Grandfather *died* in the night."

**Indirect speech:** Namitha said that Grandfather *had died* in the night.

**Note:** If old man is used in place of grandfather, 'the' should be added before 'old man'.



## Rule 2

If the reporting verb is in the present tense, the tenses in the Direct Speech do not change when it is converted to Indirect Speech.

*Let us take the examples from Rule 1.*

A. **Direct Speech:** The patient says, "I am tired".

**Indirect Speech:** The patient says he* is tired.

[*Here 'she' may also be used, as the gender is not specified]

B. **Direct Speech:** The nurse said, "Matron is supervising the junior nurses".

This has Present Continuous Tense. When this is retained, we get,

**Indirect Speech:** The nurse *has just* said that matron *is supervising* the junior nurses.

C. **Direct speech:** The teacher said, *"I have finished* the syllabus".

This has Present Perfect Tense. When this is retained, we get,

**Indirect Speech:** The teacher says she* has finished the syllabus.

[*Here 'he' may also be used, as the gender is not specified].

## Rule 3

While writing the indirect speech the pronouns in the Direct Speech are changed, where necessary.

*Example:* **Direct Speech:** Nadeem said to me, "I don't want to talk to you".

**Indirect Speech:** Nadeem said he didn't want to talk to me.

**Direct Speech:** Rehana said to Khan, "I don't believe you".

**Indirect Speech:** Rehana said she didn't believe him.

**Direct Speech:** I told him, "I don't trust you".

**Indirect Speech:** I said I didn't trust him.

(Here I told him that I don't/didn't trust him is wrong in usage. Most Asian Students make this mistake while talking it sounds right sometimes but not always.

## Rule 4

When we find words expressing nearness in the time or place in a Direct Speech, they are generally changed into words expressing distance in the Indirect Speech.

The list of such changes is given below.

- *Now* becomes *then*
- *Here* becomes *there*
- *Ago* becomes *before*
- *Thus* becomes *so*
- *Today* becomes *that day*
- *Tomorrow* becomes *the next day*
- *Yesterday* becomes *the day before*
- *Last night* becomes *the night before*

- *This* becomes *that*
- *These* becomes *those*

Let us take an example sentence to see how this works.

**Direct Speech:** John said, " I am happy to be *here this* evening".

**Indirect Speech:** John said that he was happy/glad to be *there that* evening.

## *Rule 5*

If in the Direct Speech, interrogative word is used, it is changed in the Indirect Speech by using verbs like, *asked, inquired*. If there is no interrogative word *whether* or *if* are used while writing the indirect speech.

**Example:**

**Direct Speech:** The mother asked the nurse, "When will you give the injection"?

**Indirect Speech:** The mother asked the nurse when would she give the injection.

**Direct Speech:** "Where do you live"?, asked the doctor.

**Indirect speech:** The doctor enquired where I lived.

**Direct speech:** The hostel warden said to us, "Where are you going"?

**Indirect speech:** The hostel warden enquired where we were going.

**Direct speech:** She said "Will you listen to such a girl"?

**Indirect speech:** She asked them whether they would listen to such a girl.

## *Rule 6*

When the Direct Speech contains commands and requests, the Indirect Speech has some Verb expressing command or request, and the imperative mood is changed into the Infinitive.

**Direct Speech:** Heba said to Rohan, "Go away"

**Indirect Speech:** Heba ordered Rohan to go away.

**Direct Speech:**

The peon said to Kamal, "Please wait here till I return"

The peon requested Kamal to wait there till he returned.

[Notice that all the different changes, tense, pronoun, time, place, are seen here clearly].

**Direct Speech:** "Send the first patient," said the consulting surgeon.

**Indirect Speech:** The consulting surgeon commanded them to call the first patient.

**Direct Speech:** She shouted, "Let me go".

**Indirect Speech:** She shouted to them to let her go.



## *Rule 7*

When the Direct Speech has exclamations and wishes, the Indirect Speech is written or expressed by some verb expressing *exclamation* or *wish.*

**Direct Speech:** She said, "Alas! I am bankrupt".

**Indirect Speech:** She exclaimed sadly that she was bankrupt.

**Direct Speech:** Meena said," How clever I am"!

**Indirect Speech:** Meena exclaimed that she was very clever.

**Direct Speech:** The board said, "Bravo! You all have done well".

**Indirect Speech**: The board (members of a committee) applauded them, saying that they had done well.

Now try the exercises given below to clear any confusion you may have with Direct and Indirect Speech.

## Exercises

**I . Write the following sentences in Indirect Speech:**

1. Doctor Satya said to me, "I have often told you to take your medicines on time".

2. "You have all done it very badly!" remarked the lecturers.

3. "Open your mouth, and put out your tongue" instructed Dr Suresh.

4. "What do you want?" she said to her.

5. Ananya said, "How's your mother?"

6. The poor woman exclaimed, "Will none of you help me?"

7. "Which way did he go?" asked Vaibhav.

8. Aladin said to the magician, "What have I done to deserve this fate?"

9. "Teach me a new melody," said young Sandra to the music teacher.

10. "Don't you know the way home?" she asked.

11. "Which is the proper way to answer this question, mother?" the girl enquired.

12. They said, "Who are you, madam, and what do you want?"

_______________________________________________

13. "Take off your hat," the king said to the Miller.

_______________________________________________

14. "Halt!" shouted the drill sergeant to his men.

_______________________________________________

15. She said to me, "Wait until I come."

_______________________________________________

16. "Hurry up," they said to the servant, "do not waste time."

_______________________________________________

17. King Midas said, "Daughter, take my golden jug, and fetch me some water from the lake."

_______________________________________________

18. "Go to the market and fetch some vegetables," said my mother.

_______________________________________________

19. "You are a stupid fellow!" he angrily remarked.

_______________________________________________

20. She said, "Oh! that's a nuisance."

_______________________________________________

21. They said, "How cruel of him!"

_______________________________________________

22. Ankith said, "What a pity you did not come!"

_______________________________________________

23. The priest said, "We are all sinners."

_______________________________________________

24. Ramya said, "I shall go as soon as it is possible."

25. Prakash said, "Europe is a beautiful place to visit."

You will many a time come across many types of situations which would be reported to others later. Such times you would be talking in Indirect Speech for a lengthy time. How do you go about it? Here are a few situations. Convert them into reported speech.

**II. Convert the following conversations into Indirect Speech. As these are conversations with descriptions, the answers have to be written in paragraphs.**

1. The trekker said, "Can you tell me the way to the nearest village shop?" "Yes", said the villagers; "Do you want one in which you can have food to eat?" "No", replied the trekker. "I only want to buy some biscuits and sweets." "Walk down this trail and turn left when you see a temple under the huge banyan tree. Cross the tree and go straight till you come to a well. Turn to your left and you will see the village shop," said the villager.



As a nurse you will be dealing with children. It becomes very important for you to understand the language used by children especially when they talk in English. Here is a sample of how young children speak. Let's see if you can understand their talk and convert it into Indirect Speech.

2. This is Nottis Ergunt. We arh overtenn klub. Their will, be a meating tomorrough afternun of people over, tenn to gett up an overtenn, klub ennyone, overtenn kan kum not annimuls. Prezidant will make a speach people, that interrupp him will, be chuckd out".

Now you are ready to face the challenge of writing a report. Report writing comes up ahead. At this point you may have the question "Is it possible to convert Indirect Speech to Direct Speech?" Yes. It is possible. Since, this conversion is not used in any aspect of your syllabus, we have not covered it here. Undergraduates studying English literature study it as it helps in various forms of writing. Let us move to the next topic.

# Part III

- Punctuation Marks
- Paragraph Writing
- Letter Writing

Chapter 15

# Punctuation Marks

The word punctuation is derived from the Latin word '*punctum*', which means a point. Thus the term Punctuation means the right use of putting in Points or Stops in writing. Stops in writing do not mean a full stop only.

The list of points or stops in writing are:

1. Full stop or period ( . )
2. Comma ( , )
3. Semicolon ( ; )
4. Colon ( : )
5. Interrogation mark ( ? )
6. Exclamation mark ( ! )
7. Dash ( ___ )
8. Hyphen ( - )
9. Parentheses or brackets ( )
10. Apostrophe ( ' )
11. Inverted Commas or Quotation Marks ( " " )
12. Capital letters ( ABCD )

Let us now try to understand all the functions done by these punctuation marks.

## Full Stop or Period ( . )

This is denoted by the dot. This shows the completion of a sentence.

***Uses***

i. To mark the end of a sentence; as

The doctor is doing the rounds.

ii. To mark abbreviations and initials; as

Mr., Mrs., A.V. Hume, B.A., B.Sc.,

iii. Serve as decimal points for numbers; as

21.4%, 15.95

> ***Note:*** If a sentence comes to an end with an abbreviation, no second Period (.) is necessary.



## Comma ( , )

This represents the shortest pause, while reading or writing.

***Used in***

i. separating a series of words or ideas in the same sentence.

***Example:*** Nurse Vidya wrote her notes neatly, quickly and correctly.

We went to England, France, Germany and Greece this summer.

ii. separating each pair of words connected by 'and'.

***Example:*** They are poor and honest, cheerful and hardworking.

Rich and poor, wise and foolish, smart and dumb must all die.

iii. joining compound sentences linked by and, but, or, for nor, yet and sometimes 'so'.

***Example:*** "The more we earn, the less we seem to care, for money does not bring the satisfaction we thought it would", said Dr Ismail.

It was strong, yet it was not unpleasant.

Blessed are the meek, for they shall inherit the earth.

iv. joining short sentences in series.

***Example:*** We can, we will, we must.

v. a sentence when an interjection is introduced, it is set off by a comma.

*Example:* Oh, is that the final diagnosis?

vi. when a direct address introduces a sentence, it is set off by a comma.

*Example:* Maria, you've done a great job.

vii. To emphasize a contrast or to give added emphasis to a particular word, phrase or clause.

*Example:* The more embroidery on a dress, the higher the price.

The more demanding a course, the longer hours one has to study.

viii. To increase the readability of addresses, place names, dates, statistics and measurement and to serve other conventional purpose.

*Example:*
a. September 3, 2008
b. 18, 695
c. No. 69, 37th Cross, Jayanagar, Bangalore - 560069, India
d. February 18, 2018, is his retirement
e. Phillip. R. Evans, MD

ix. Salutations and complimentary close in informal letters;

a. Dear Janet,

b. Sincerely,

c. Regards,

## Semi-colon ( ; )

This shows a pause of greater importance than that shown by the comma. It is like a blinking red traffic light at an intersection. It signals a brief but definite stop.

***Used***

a. to separate two or more main clauses if they are closely connected in meaning. Like,

i. Our classes were cancelled; we students went for a movie.

ii. The child vomited; nurse Maria calmed the child as she cleaned the child.

Since the semicolon is as good as a full stop, it is possible to rewrite the above examples using a full-stop instead of a semicolon. Like,

i. Our classes were cancelled. We students went for a movie.

ii. The child vomited. Nurse Maria calmed the child as she cleaned the child.

But here, the full stop breaks the line of thought by separating the ideas which are closely linked. Therefore the semicolon, is used as the ides are retained.

b. To separate items in a list which are more in number and already have commas. Like,

   i. The UNICEF medical team consisted of Dr Aliya from India; Dr Mehnaz from Kuwait; Dr Paulette from Britain and Dr Jacque Thom from France.

   ii. On the tray were scalpels, scissors and forceps; needles and suture; retractors, gloves and swabs; sterilised and ready for use.

c. To show the relationship between the main clauses more plain.

   This is when the semi-colon is followed by a conjunctive adverb, like:

   i. She knew she would faint at the sight of blood; all the same she watched the matron draw the blood sample from her son's hand.



## Colon ( : )

This is termed a more complete pause than that expressed by the semicolon. It is usually used with a dash.

It is used

a. to introduce a quotation. Like–

   i. Swami Vivekananda says: "Awake, rise and stop not till your goal is reached."

b. to introduce a list or an enumeration of items or examples. Like–

   ii. Mother gave the grocer a list of things she wanted. The list is here:

| Grocery list: | Rice | – | 10 kgs |
|---|---|---|---|
| | Flour | – | 1 kg |

| | | |
|---|---|---|
| Butter | – | 500 gms |
| Margarine | – | 500 gms |
| Custard powder | – | 1 packet |
| Beans | – | 1 kg |

c. to indicate that an explanation or elaboration of a general statement will follow.

*Example:*

i. Tuberculosis at one time was a great killer: It killed thirty thousand a year.

ii. Sister Yogita is an ideal social worker: Brave, honest, reliable and trustworthy.

d. To mark conventional separations like

i. Hours from minutes — 6:45 am

ii. Rhymes or related terms — walk: balk,
red: white

iii. Chapter from verse in religious texts

Samuel 5 : 8
Daniel 7 : 6

iv. Volume from page, like — III : 86

v. Title from subtitle, like — Kenneth Anderson: a collection of short stories

vi. Introductory tags, like — From left to right:Dr Malini, Dr Vidya, Matron Stella.

vii. Numerals in ratio, like — 3:9, 4:10

viii. Place from Publisher (this is sometimes found in bibliographies and thesis works)

London: Palmer Mary and Churchill Brown.

## Interrogation Mark ( ? )

This is also called as the question mark.

a. An interrogation mark ends a sentence asking a direct question. Like–

i. Where is the needle?

ii. Which way should we go to reach the maternity ward?

iii. When was Penicillin discovered?

b. Sometimes a question mark is used to make an ironic commentary.

*Example:* The newspapers reported that unarmed (?) people were present at the religious meeting.

c. This is used after a question within quotation marks:

Dr Verma asked the patient, 'Does it pain here? Around the navel?'

d. This is used after a 'tag' question. Like–

You saw the accident happen, didn't you?

> ***Note:*** We do not use a question mark to end an indirect question like, She asked me if my nursing notes were completed.



## Exclamation Mark ( ! )

This is used to

a. Show emotions in a word, phrase or a sentence.
Like–

i. Hurrah!

ii. Alas! My child is no more.

iii. What a lovely party!

b. Show charged feelings,

Like–

i. Get lost! I never want to see you again!

ii. We should be careful in not overusing this.

## Dash ( — )

This is used to–

i. show an abrupt stop or change of thoughts. Like–

If my grand-father were alive— but why talk of the past?

If the rules had not changed—why talk of what is not to be?

ii. continue a scattered subject like,

Teachers, parents, friends—all scolded him.

iii. sometimes used to achieve suspense, or anticlimax like,

There is somebody in his life—himself.

## Hyphen ( - )

This is a shorter line than the Dash (—).

i. It is used to connect the parts of a compound word. Like–

Passer-by

Chief-of-Army

Grand-father

Pea-cock

ii. Used when two or more words modifying a noun and used as a single adjective, like

She is a soft-spoken, well-mannered doctor.

iii. Used in words made up of a prefix and a proper noun.

*Example:* He is anti-American.

The crowd is pro-British.

iv. When single-letters are joined to a noun, like

T-shirt

v. When numerals from 21 onwards are written in words

twenty-one, seventy-two.

vi. To form fractions, and compounds with numbers, like

One-tenth of a minute.

One-fifth of the cake.

Two-day pass. The sailor got a two-day pass to go ashore.

Twelve-year-old

The twelve-year-old child was admitted with severe asthma.

vii. Used to divide word into syllables, like

Spon-ta-ne-ous

Com-puter



## Parenthesis or Brackets ( )

This is used:

i. to enclose explanations, changing topics while writing and interruptions to the main thought of the sentence.

*Example:* The trend indicates (see table 3) that inefficiency is increasing.

The study shows (see the chart) that protein deficiency is coming under control.

ii. to enclose numbers and letters making divisions included in the main text. Like–

The physiological changes in (a) the female of the Rhesus monkey

(b) the male of the chimpanzees

iii. to enclose phonetic transcriptions. Like–

ran (ræn)

lecture (lekt ∂)

# Punctuation Marks

## Apostrophe ( ' )

This looks like a raised comma.

Apostrophe is used

i. to show the possessive case of nouns and indefinite pronouns. In other words this punctuation mark shows that a thing belongs to someone (possessive). This is used along with s to show possession ('s).

*Example:* My mother's car is in the garage.

The car's tyre is punctured.

The patient's hand is bandaged.

That is Dr Kumar's bag.

Plural possessive is formed by adding an apostrophe to the plural of words that end in `s'. If the plural is irregular an 's' is added to the plural form.

*Example:* The men's ward is on the left.

A children's book caught the attention of the child psychologist.

Arvind attended a fathers' and sons' banquet.

ii. to show shortening or the omissions of letters.

*Is it not* becomes *isn't*

*Madam* becomes *ma'am*

*Do not* becomes *don't*

*I have* becomes *I've*

iii. to form plurals of numbers, letters, signs, abbreviations, dates and words used as words, like–

6's and 7's, the 1960's.

## Quotation Marks or Inverted Commas or Quotes (“ ”) (‘ ’)

They are called so as they are commas put in the opposite way, above the line of writing instead of along the line of writing. They are of two types; single quotes ' ' and double quotes " ".

Chapter 15

They are used

i. to identify direct quotes, like–

Kenney said, "Don't ask what your country does to you. Ask what you can do to your country."

ii. to identify spoken dialogue, like–

1. 'Now, Prof Ruchquayya will address the class', said Dr. Ali Hyder.
2. 'Please wheel the patient in', requested the old man to the nurse, showing his grandson, sitting dazed in the wheelchair.

'Will you come to the lab now?' asked Jenny.

iii. to enclose titles of stories, plays, poems, essays, articles appearing in a larger work, like–

Did you read the article 'Diabetes and the Indian people' that appeared in today's paper?

iv. to enclose a word or expression that is being defined, like–

The word 'abscess' means 'pus filled wound'.

v. to indicate the names of songs, short musical compositions, radio and TV programmes, like–

MTV's "Classic hits".

vi. to indicate or suggest irony.

*Example:*

"It was the dog that died that bit the man".

## Capital Letters

These are used

i. to begin the first word of a sentence, line of poetry a fragment written as a sentence.

*Example:* Hospitals should always be maintained clean and tidy.

ii. to identify Proper Nouns (names of people and places), initials and abbreviations.

| | | | |
|---|---|---|---|
| Bal Gangadhar Tilak | Mount Kailash | BBC | BA |
| Thomas Alva Edison | Mumbai | VOA | MSc |
| Pune University | | | |

iii. The high ranks, titles in government offices, heads of state, religious heads etc.

| | | |
|---|---|---|
| Field Marshall Verma | President Pratibha Patil | the Pope |
| Mrs Karan | the Prime Minister | |

iv. to show the names of days, months, holidays and religious days.

Thursday, May, Christmas

iv. With the names of historical events, names of historical or cultural periods, races, tribes, nationalities, languages, religions and holy books and the titles of literary works.

*Example:*

| | | |
|---|---|---|
| The Second World War, | Aryan, | The Bible |
| The Golden Age of the Cholas, | Caucasian, | The Merchant of Venice, |
| The Bhagavad-Gita, | French, | Gone with the Wind |



## Exercises

**I. Use the appropriate punctuation mark (full stop, question mark, exclamation, capital letters) with the following:**

1. danny is ill yet he refuses to see a doctor
2. they are terrified of surgery
3. caesarian operations are carried out by competent gynaecologist
4. the nurse is giving mary an injection
5. Oooh what a beautiful slide
6. the nurses of a b2 batch will be posted to the female medical ward today
7. the aids patient has lost his hope to live
8. yuck the toilets stink
9. are they afraid of dr reshma rao
10. what are you doing here asked the mother

**The following passage is usually heard in a clinic between a doctor and the patient. The quotation marks, commas, full stops, capital letters, question marks, hyphens and exclamatory marks are missing. Can you insert them?**

When the doctor called next a young woman with her six year old son entered the mother was looking worried and anxious the boy was quiet

good evening mrs shastry what is the matter asked the doctor oh dr suresh my son slipped on the wet kitchen floor fell cut his chin on the sharp edge of the cupboard door that was open it started bleeding i kept a wet cloth on the wound and quickly got him here should there be stitches is it too deep

calmly doctor suresh was cleaning the wound as the mother was narrating the incident, he examined the wound by the foucs lamp he smiled and said no need to worry the wound is not deep no need for stitches no need to give the anti-tetanus injection as he has had the Booster mrs shastry sighed in relief wow no injection cried aditya so you were keeping quiet thinking you ll have to take injection young aditya asked the doctor with a twinkle in his eye dr suresh finished putting medicine on the wound and dressed it he patted the boy and gently told him to be careful while rushing about the house

good night doctor and thank you said mrs shastry

good night mrs shastry and get him 3 days later see you young man said dr shastry

bye doctor said little aditya

**II. Supply capital letters, semicolons, dashes, hyphens, apostrophes and colons where required:**

1. didn t the doctor tell you not to eat hot food again.
2. the capitals of a few indian states are karnataka banagalore, jammu and kashmir jammu, sikkim gangtok, tamil nadu, chennai.
3. disorders due to mutant genes are Brachy dactyly, huntingon's chorea, sickle cell anaemia, phenylketonuria, red green colour blindness and haemophilia.
4. here's some good news for you you have won the competition.
5. there are thirty six nurses in this class.
6. students aren't sure when they have their exam.
7. my teacher was not just irritated he was very angry.
8. it was 1030 am. When my cousin rowena landed in delhi.

9. my advice to you is this consult with your wife before you buy that house.
10. All my grandchildren are studying in highschool
11. the fifteen year old wanted to become a high flying ceo when he grew up.
12. "they d played together in infancy," informed the grandmother to her grandchildren about their grand father and his friend.
13. we tried hard we failed.
14. the congregation started reading the psalm given in daniel 7 9.
15. there were only two things to do run or jump.
16. gloria had to learn how to manage her demanding mother in law and her hyper active child.
17. the musicals of 1960s are popular even now.
18. doctors neednt bother about the memo not going around. It ll be done by the administrative staff.
19. doctors worked hard to save mother and child they failed.
20. that is my fathers college photograph. You can see him and his cousins. They are standing left to right jack, ron, william and albert.

You are now ready for the next phase of your learning –Writing paragraphs. Punctuations are used everywhere. By changing any one of them, either a misunderstanding or a hilarious situation can be created.

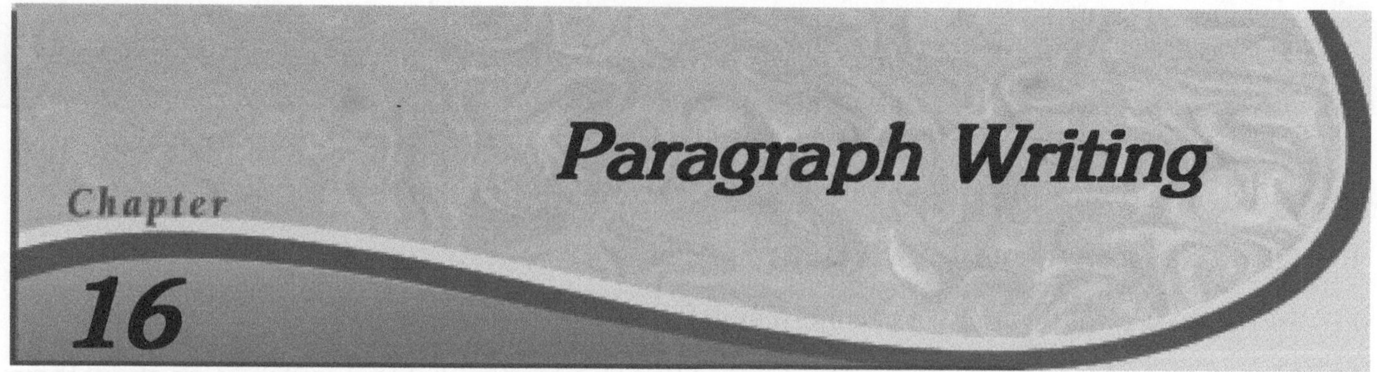


When we see any printed matter, or written matter, we see that some lines are grouped together. Many such lines are grouped together in reports, essays, newspapers and your own notes. These lines grouped together usually have a common idea. Such sentences which are grouped together in a piece of writing is called a paragraph.

The first line of every paragraph will be slightly indented to the right. Paragraphs are in chapters, essays and other prose compositions. This is done to make reading easier. The beginning of a new paragraph shows change of topic or a step in the development of an argument or of a story.

***Definition:*** A paragraph is a number of sentences grouped together and relating to one topic.

OR

A group of related sentences that develop a single point is called a **paragraph**.

There is no rule as to the length of a paragraph. They may be long or short according to the necessity of the subject chosen.

A paragraph is different from the stanzas of a poem. Stanzas are usually of the same length and pattern. But paragraphs are long or short according to the amount of matter to be expressed.

So, now let us check some paragraphs.

1. Without a clock everything would be in a dreadful mess. Doctors and Nurses have to work wasting no time. It was John Harrison who made the clock wheels out of wood. The sailor needs the clock more than anyone else.

2. A dog is a man's best friend, but it cannot talk. It is believed that from pre-historic times dogs were domesticated. There are many varieties of dogs. Dogs usually come in various sizes. Wolves are believed to be the ancestors of dogs. Wolves live in packs and have a leader. But, black, white, brown, grey happen to be the standard dog colours. The various shades in these colours are found on the various varieties of dogs. Cold country dogs are found to have more hair.

3. Mango is the king of fruits. It is one of the most versatile fruits with its own special aroma, fragrance and texture. Green or ripe, it can be used in a number of dishes and very imaginatively too. The mango is replete with all the vital vitamins you require such as vitamin 'B', 'C', calcium, carotene, protein, iron and fiber. Both green and ripe mangoes are great to look at and a delight for the palate. Many exotic dishes can be created with the pulp of ripe mangoes, as also with green mangoes.

Now, let us analyse these paragraphs.

**The first paragraph** is about clock and time. If you read the paragraph carefully you will notice that although all the four sentences are grammatically correct and also convey meaning in isolation they do not combine together to make a good paragraph. You will feel that something is missing.

Observe the paragraph closely. The first sentence deals with the necessity of having a clock. The reader naturally expects this idea to continue in the second. But the second sentence neither supports nor illustrates that idea. Again the third sentence is not related to the second, but tells us about the inventor of the clock. The fourth sentence though loosely related to the first, does not come as a natural sequence to the third. Thus, this piece of writing does not have a single controlling idea, i.e., a central idea and hence, it cannot be considered a paragraph.

**Paragraph (2)** reads better than **(1)**. The first sentence states that a dog is man's best friend, but it cannot talk. The second sentence develops this idea—it is believed that from pre-historic times dogs were domesticated. The third sentence tells about variety of dogs. Fourth sentence tells about their sizes.

This paragraph has a single controlling idea namely the dog. But the fifth and sixth sentences say more about the wolves than the dog. Naturally, the reader is left wondering whether the paragraph has more than one central idea. In other words, another idea about the wolf disturbs the unity of the paragraph.

**Now look at paragraph** (3). The paragraph begins with the controlling idea, namely the Mango is the king of fruits. Sentence (2) and (3) contribute to this idea stating how its properties are and its uses. Sentences (4) and (5) illustrate the nutritional value of mango and the ways in which it can be used to prepare dishes.

Thus, the paragraph has–

i. A central idea (main idea), and

ii. The idea is completely developed.

The central idea is stated in a sentence as can be seen from paragraph (3) i.e., "**Mango is the king of fruits**." This sentence is called as the **Topic sentence**. The Topic sentence may occur in the beginning, in the middle or at the end of the paragraph. Sometimes the topic sentence may not be clearly stated but only implied.

So we realise that there are certain rules to be followed while writing a paragraph.

This brings us to the principles of paragraph structure. Paragraph (3) follows all the principles. Thus, it reads well.

There are three principles:

1. Unity
2. Order
3. Variety



1. *Unity:* This is the most important principle to be followed while constructing a paragraph. Every sentence deals with one thought. Same way, every paragraph must deal with ***one topic or idea.*** While writing an essay or report, for example, every heading and every sub-heading should have its own paragraph to itself. Every sentence in the paragraph must be closely connected with the main topic of the paragraph. The *Topical sentence or the key-sentence* opens the subject to be dealt within the paragraph.
2. *Order:* This is logical sequence of thought or development of the subject. Points must be put in the order of their occurrence and all ideas must be connected with the main idea. The points must be arranged according to their importance. Two or three sentences support the main idea and help in developing it. They are called ***supporting sentences***. In this regard we must remember that the first and last sentences in the paragraph are the most important sentences. The first sentence is usually the topic sentence, should catch the interest of the reader and the last sentence should satisfy the interest generated. The topic sentence states the topic (subject or title)– a fact, a statement or a proposition. The last sentence should bring the whole paragraph on the topic chosen to a conclusion.
3. *Variety:* This means that the length of the paragraphs in an essay, report or writing should be of different lengths. This breaks the monotony. The reader does not get bored.

So in all, we can say that a good paragraph requires the following elements.

1. Unity
2. A good topical sentence
3. Logical sequence of thought
4. Variety, and
5. A full and rounded final sentence in conclusion.

Before confusion occurs, let us put these points in the form of a flow chart. This will help for easy remembrance.

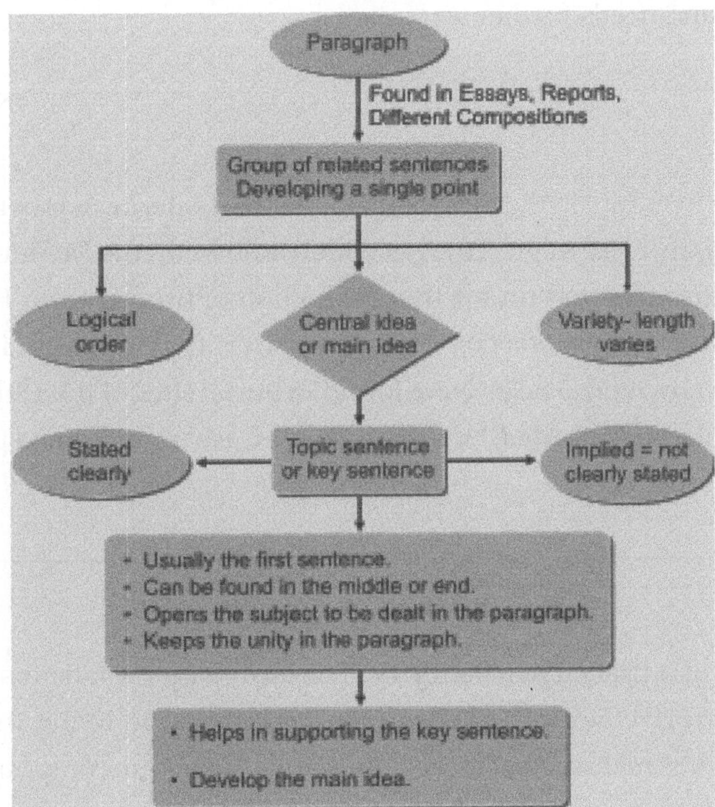


## Exercises

**I. Some paragraphs are given here. Identify the Topic or key sentence.**

Say whether it is stated or implied.

1. The earth is enclosed in a layer of air, called the atmosphere. This extends upwards approximately two hundred miles. This atmosphere, is a mixture of gases. This gets thinner, or less dense, as height increases, and there is hardly any at all fifty to sixty miles up. It is the movement of air within the atmosphere which brings different weather conditions.

   **Topic sentence** ________________________________________

   Implied/stated

2. To test for colour fastness, soak each fabric individually in a basin of very warm water for 15 minutes. Swish the fabric around and then wring it out. If the water remains clear, then the fabric is colour-fast. It may be tossed into the washing machine for preshrinking. If the water is discoloured, the fabric fails the test and needs further treatment.

   **Topic sentence** ________________________________________

   Implied/stated

3. Tin typically occurs in nature in the form of the mineral cassiterite. It is believed that man discovered tin about 6-6.5 thousand years ago. Tin was widely known in the Mediterranean countries, Persia, and India. Egyptians imported tin for the production of bronze from Persia. In his book *Ancient Egyptian Materials and Their production*, A. Lukas writes that although in Egypt tin ores were not known, the oldest known tin articles were found in burial sites of the 18th dynasty. Tin was known not only in the countries of the Mediterranean; Julius Caesar mentioned production of tin in central regions of Britain.

   **Topic sentence** ________________________________________

   Implied/stated

4. Organic Chemistry is a branch of Chemistry. The term Organic Chemistry was originally used to describe scientific work concerning substances to be found in living things such as animals and plants. However, it was realised that most of these substances are compounds of the element carbon, and organic chemistry now means the chemistry of the very large number of the compounds of carbon.

   **Topic sentence** ________________________________________

   Implied/stated

5. According to medical studies, an inadequate protein intake in the diet often leads to protein calorie malnutrition or PCM. PCM is also called protein energy malnutrition or PEM. One such deficiency is called kwashiorkor.

This disease of infants and young children is caused by severe protein deficiency. Millions of babies in Asia including India, Africa and Latin America suffer from this deficiency disease. It is caused when instead of their mother's milk, they take mainly a carbohydrate diet that too in an inadequate amount. The children suffering from kwashiorkor become irritable, miserable, cease to grow and lose weight. The skin becomes scaly, dark and shows ugly cracks. Hair takes on a reddish colour. The body swells due to water retention in the cells (oedema): Belly protrudes and limbs become thin and bony. Brain development and mental capacities are retarded. The liver too is damaged and the child often dies before the age of five. Such children also become increasingly susceptible to various infections.

On account of poverty in Asia and Africa many cases of kwashiorkor are neglected. In the absence of mother's milk, a protein-rich diet obtained from animals or from soya bean, or a mixture of corn, cotton-seed, yeast and leaf-meal or a combination of wheat, gram, peanuts and jaggery, can effectively cure this African named disease.

**Topic sentence** ________________________________

Implied/stated

6. The batting is the layer between the top and the bottom of the quilt. The batting adds the warmth and weight and makes the quilting stitches more than simple stitches on a flat surface.

If you were to examine several old quilts, you would find more than one type of batting. Cotton was surely the most common, complete with seeds. It is not unusual to find an old woollen blanket put to good use between quilt top and quilt backing. Other "Quilts" were made by layering fabrics to create a heavy quilt top and had no batting or quilting stitches at all.

**Topic sentence** ________________________________

Implied/stated

7. Trekking is a hobby pursued by a few people. It is walking for miles together either in a forest, or on a mountain, or along the coastline. Some daring individuals walk across a desert too. While going on a trek, required clothing, food, water and basic medicines are packed in a backpack and carried by each individual. A trek can be for a day or go on for 15-20 days. It all depends on the route and

the final destination the group or the individual decides on. A sleeping bag is carried by every individual if the trek lasts for more than one day. Trekking can be undertaken by people of all ages.

**Topic sentence** ______________________________

Implied/stated

8. In 1796, Dr Edward Jenner inoculated a boy against the dreaded disease of smallpox which killed many thousands of people. He used a vaccine made from the cow-pox sores of a milkmaid. The boy caught the lesser disease of cow-pox and recovered but, when later inoculated with smallpox itself; he showed no signs of catching it. The practice of vaccination, as it came to be called, was quickly adopted throughout the western world. By 1801 at least one hundred thousand persons had been vaccinated in England.

**Topic sentence** ______________________________

Implied/stated



**II. Now let us see if you can show the supporting sentences in the above paragraphs. One is done for you.**

1. According to medical studies, an inadequate protein intake in the diet often leads to protein calorie malnutrition or PCM. PCM is also called protein energy malnutrition or PEM. One such deficiency is called Kwashiorkor. This disease of infants and young children is caused by severe protein deficiency. Millions of babies in Asia including India, Africa and Latin America suffer from this deficiency disease. It is caused when instead of their mother's milk, they take mainly a carbohydrate diet that too in an inadequate amount. The children suffering from kwashiorkor become irritable, miserable, cease to grow and lose weight.

**Topic sentence**

*Millions of babies in Asia including India, Africa and Latin America suffer from this deficiency disease*

1. Supporting sentence: *This disease of infants and young children is caused by severe protein deficiency.*
2. Supporting sentences are:

______________________________

______________________________

3. Supporting sentences are:

______________________________

______________________________

4. Supporting sentences are:

_______________________________________________

_______________________________________________

5. Supporting sentences are:

_______________________________________________

_______________________________________________

6. Supporting sentences are:

_______________________________________________

_______________________________________________

7. Supporting sentences are:

_______________________________________________

_______________________________________________

8. Supporting sentences are:

_______________________________________________

_______________________________________________



**II. Here are some more paragraphs. Identify the Topic Sentence and the Supporting Sentences.**

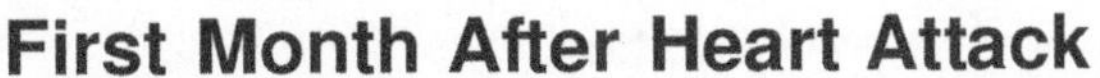

## First Month After Heart Attack

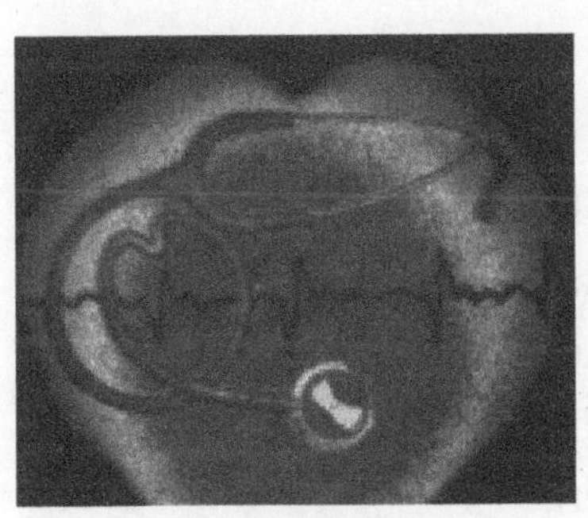

People who survive heart attack are at much higher risk of sudden cardiac death in the next 30 days, researches have found. The findings, which appeared in the Journal of the American Medical Association, suggest that doctors need to closely supervise patients in the month after a heart attack. The patients also need to be alert to signs of trouble. "The first month after a heart attack can be envisioned as a period of healing with heart tissue remodeling, which conceptually is associated with a propensity to experience sudden death", one of the authors, Dr Veronique. L Roger of the Mayo clinic in Rochester, said in an e-mail message. Researchers found that the first month after a heart is crucial. The rate of sudden cardiac death was 1.2%. This is about four times the risk that would have been expected in the general population, once age and sex were taken into account.

**Topic Sentence:**

Supporting Sentences:

1. ______________________________

2. ______________________________

## Tea Bags

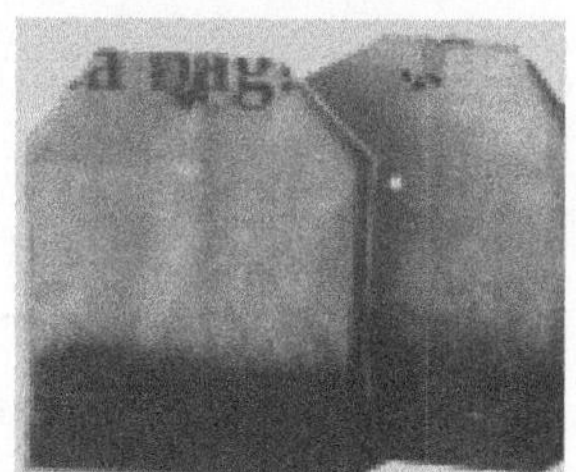


It is 104 years since the first tea bag was delivered. The first one was tea delivered in a silk sachet. Mass commercial production of paper tea bags didn't start until the 1950s.

Tea bag tea tastes different from tea pot tea. 96% of households world wide now use tea bags. The old brew-up principal of one teaspoon per cup and one for the pot, tea bags are more economical. Can we really hang tea bags up on a line, dry them and reuse them? The answer surprisingly is yes, if you use two per cup. Best not to tell important guests, though. Right?!

**Topic Sentence:**

Supporting Sentences:

3. ______________________________

4. ______________________________

## Sweet Nothings

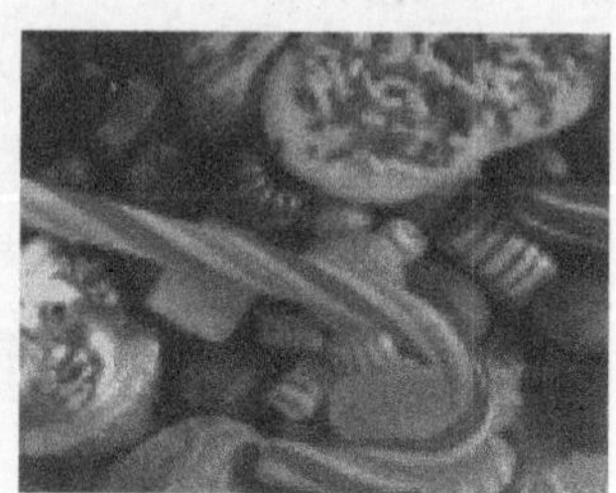

India is the diabetes capital of the world. And Indian women have a 11-fold risk of developing diabetes during pregnancy when compared to Caucasian or Western women. According to latest medical studies, one of seven pregnant women has diabetes in urban India! The Diabetes in Pregnancy Study Group, India (DIPSI) recommends diabetic screening for all pregnant women. Gestational diabetes is a type of diabetes that occurs in the 2nd and 3rd trimesters of pregnancy. At this time there is an increase in placental hormones. Screening for gestational diabetes is a must for all pregnant women.

**Topic Sentence:**

Supporting Sentences:

1. ______________________________

2. ______________________________

## Babies and Coincidences

Once in a hospital three men were sitting in the waiting room of a hospital. A nurse came from the labour room and walked over to the first man. Looking at him, she said, "congratulations. You 're the father of twins." "What a coincidence," he said, "I work for Twin Town Bank." A little while later, the nurse came out to congratulate the Second man. "You are the proud father of triplets" she said. The new dad said, "That's funny, I work for AAA." Both the new fathers looked at each other and started talking about pleasant coincidences. At this, the third man who was also expecting news jumped up a look of terror on his face. He ran out of the waiting room. The Nurse quickly called out "Sir, where are you going?" The man yelled, "I work for Seven Up!"

**Topic Sentence:**

Supporting Sentences:

1. ______________________________

2. ______________________________

After all these, we come to another interesting portion. Skimming, scanning and reading.

## Reading Strategies

Usually every student who learns English asks "why should I **Read?**" The answers are many and varied. Some of the answers may not be pleasant to hear for a student still struggling to learn English. This brings us to the next question "why should I read only in English?" The answer to this is "No need to read only in English. Read all materials possible in every language you know." This brings us back to the first question "why Read?"

First and foremost, you as a nursing student need to read the instructions written by the doctor about a patient. This helps in the healing process. Next you need to read and understand your text. books and notes to get your Graduation Certificate to become a nurse. After this, you may be called upon to read medical files of your near and dear ones and explain to them in simple words about their predicaments. Then you have to read letters from home, friends, formal letters, in your work place. After this, you have to read newspapers advertising job vacancies and opportunities. Later when you are a parent yourself, you will be required to read aloud to your child/children and teach them skills to develop their personalities.

All along you cannot stop updating your knowledge of new discoveries, inventions, procedures, information in the vast field of medicine.

The list of answers for this question is endless. I hope you are convinced of the necessity to read regardless of the language.

Now to tackle the point "Reading in English—is it a necessity?"

It is a necessity as English is an international language. Text books in the field of medicine and other technological fields are in English. Most of the internet, media, libraries and research data are in English. Thus it is necessary to improve one's skill in reading in English.

Everybody reads at their own speed based on how quickly they can understand the printed word. But, when you are working in a hospital, or reading all the textbooks you have or when you read a newspaper or go shopping for the groceries, you need to be very quick. This is when you require Reading Strategies.

These are skimming, scanning and drawing inferences.

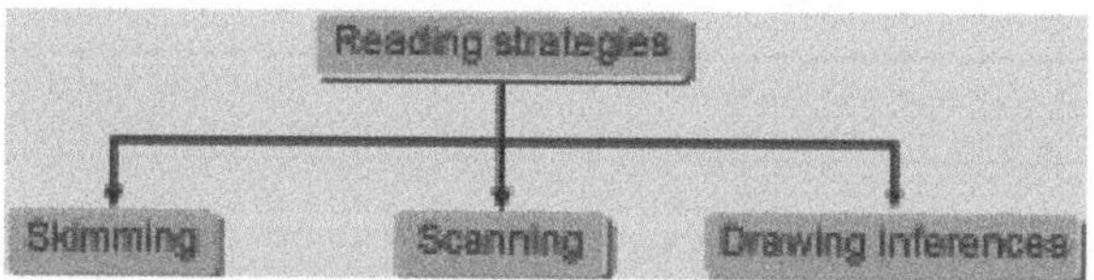


## Skimming

This means to read something quickly in order to find a particular point or the main points. Sometimes it is useful for you to be able to get the overall idea of a paragraph or passage.

- What is the paragraph or passage about?
- What kind of information does it include?
- Where is the important point in the information that I am reading?
- What type of passage/information is it? (Is it a letter? Short-story? Consumer information? An essay? A set of instructions?)

It is helpful to be able to answer these questions to decide whether you want to read the matter in front of you in more detail. This helps you to read better. This helps you to know what to expect.

This skill is called **Skimming**.

How does one **do** this? Following are the ways in which you can skim through any written material.

- Look at the title.
- Then notice the differences in print, size of the letters.
- Notice colours if any used.
- Next look at some of the important words, especially nouns and verbs.
- Try to see if you can answer the last question asked above.

The point is to read quickly, not to look carefully at every word.

## Exercise

**To help you understand this skill here is a small exercise. Read the following short passages (1-8). Mark 1 to 8 as appropriate in the space provided at the end of them.**

1.

London,

9th August 2009

Dear Charlotte,

It is with pleasure I write to you. I am expecting my first child six months from now. Isn't this wonderful?! After all the years of tests and prayers I had given up hope. To get this news now, when I least expected this…

To become a mother at 35! I am thrilled and scared at the same time. What if I do something wrong? What if this turns out to be a dream?

Julian is practical. He assures me this is no dream.

Would you be able to come over for a week or two and help me out?

Your presence is all I require.

Looking forward for a favourable reply and seeing you here.

Your thrilled cousin,

**Lauren**

2. To: All the Class Teachers

   From: The Principal, Prof.Iyer

   Date: 8 April 2009

   *Re: Exam Results*

   All the class teachers are informed to come with the details of the marks scored by the students in the classes assigned to them in the academic Year 2007-2008. Discussion regarding their performances and steps to be taken for improving them will be held on 9th April in the board-room at 10 a.m.

3. **Books and Reading**

   Happy is the person who acquires the habit of reading when one is young. One has secured a life-long source of pleasure, instruction and inspiration. So long as one has one's beloved books, one need never feel lonely. One always has a pleasant occupation of leisure moments, so that one need never feel bored. He/She is the possessor of wealth more precious than gold....



4. Twinkle, twinkle little star
   How I wonder what you are?
   Up above the world so high
   Like a diamond in the sky!

5. **Waggy the Cute Little Dog**

"Waggy come here" shouted Smitha. The moment she called him, yelping happily, wagging his tail fast, he jumped at her. Smitha started giggling in spite of her anger. Waggy was licking her hands, her legs, with his cool wet tongue and rolled over onto his back-all the four legs in the air, his white stomach ready to be tickled. He put his tongue to a side and twinkled his eyes at his young mistress. Looking at him and the pink tongue lolling out, Smitha forgot her anger, and started laughing.

She bent down and started tickling his stomach saying "You little rascal, you made me forget why I wanted to scold you. You tiny tanker....".

Waggy quickly rolled over and said "woof".

"You do understand all that I tell you. You are an intelligent dog. Now what did I want to punish you for?" wondered Smitha aloud.

6. **Chinese Noodles**

Serves 6-8

8 oz Chinese egg noodles.

Boiling water

3 tablespoons bottled chili sauce.

Place the noodles in a large pan of boiling salted water, cook for one minute. Turn off the heat and leave to stand for 4 minutes , by which time the noodles should be tender. Drain well and serve sprinkled with chili sauce.

7. April 16 1994.

Today is my birthday. But what a day! Physics exam. That too my finals. Last year in college. Yet I can't enjoy. Tomorrow is Paper IV Physics. Today it is Paper III Physics. Mama gave me a beautiful book. Sis gave me a poster. Pa gave Rs 500! Good start. But the exam tension began. Hope all will remember to wish me in college, after the paper is over today.

8. GIRL: Len darling, you are free (she embraces him) isn't it wonderful? They're trying to keep me out. Darling it's been awful. I've been nearly crazy.

- ROMAINE (with sudden violent harshness) Leonard- who –is-this girl!
- GIRL (to ROMAINE defiantly) I'm Len's girl. I know all about you.

You're not his wife. Never have been. (She crosses to right of ROMAINE) you're years older than him, and you just got hold of him—and you've done your best to hang him. But that's all over now. (She turns to Len) We'll go abroad like you said, on one of your cruises—to all those grand places. We'll have a wonderful time.

___ A diary entry

___ A memo

___ Part of a short story

___ Part of an essay

___ A letter

___ A poem

___ A recipe

___ Part of a drama

## Scanning

This means to look quickly through something written or printed in order to find specific details.

To do this you must pay close attention to words or numbers or both in the material in front of you, like, a scoreboard, or a time-table, BHT, train and bus and plane time-tables, written matter on packets etcetera.

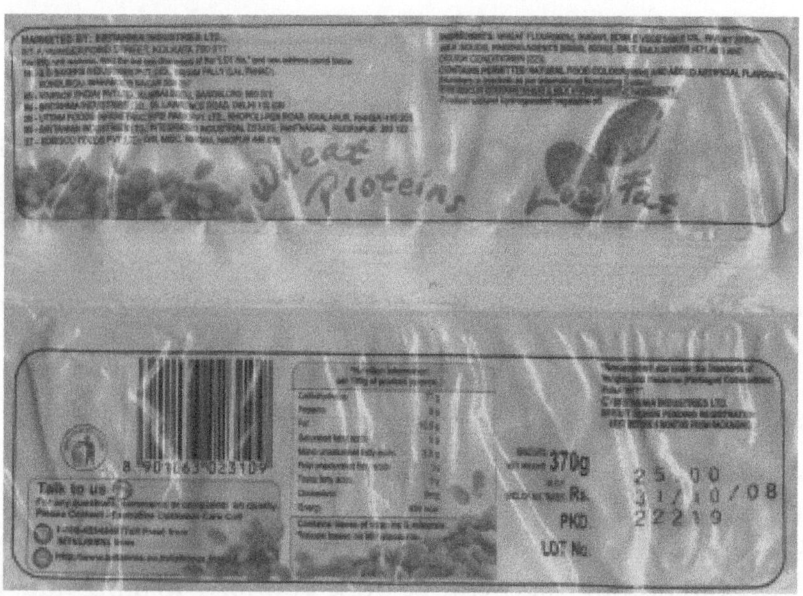


## Exercise

**Robert has purchased a packet of Marie biscuits. The following information is given on the packet.**

i. What is the date of packaging?

______________________________

ii. What is the amount of carbohydrates present in 100 g of this product?

______________________________

iii. Has the manufacturer given his web-site address?

______________________________________________

iv. Name the ingredients used in the product

______________________________________________

v. Is the shelf life given on the packet

______________________________________________

vi. What is the price of the product?

______________________________________________

## COMPREHENSION EXERCISES

Here are some Comprehension Passages. Read them as quickly as you can and answer the questions given below each. This helps you in understanding the material in front of you and hones your speed reading skill.

### Bacteria and Disease

Although the microscope had been greatly improved, little progress was made in study of bacteria following its discovery by Leeuwenhoek in 1683.

The next big step forward came in the early 19th century. The French chemist, Louis Pasteur, the most outstanding 19th century biologist, was asked by brewers to find out why bear and wine sometimes turned sour. He discovered that the souring was caused by the presence of tiny micro-organisms. He came to the conclusion that these organisms were always present in the air, and proved it by many experiments. He used various flasks and found that the contents of the sealed flasks were not affected by the germs. By heating the infected liquids for a certain length of time; he killed the air-borne bacteria. This later led to the *'pasteurization'* of milk; a process which continues today.



Pasteur next turned his attention to animal diseases, particularly of sheep and poultry. He was able to show that many of these were due to bacteria which were carried from one animal to another through the air. He believed that many human diseases could be passed from one person to another in the same way, a belief that was later to be proved correct.

Pasteur's experiments led to new science—the science of bacteriology.

1. When was bacteria discovered by Leeuwenhoek?

   ______________________________

2. Louis Pasteur was a biologist. True or false?

   ______________________________

3. How did beer and wine sometimes turn sour?

   ______________________________

4. What is 'pasteurization' of milk?

   ______________________________

5. Has micro-organisms got to do anything with wine turning sour?

_______________

6. What causes diseases in sheep and poultry?

_______________

7. Is air the carrier of bacteria?

_______________

8. Haw are diseases spread in humans?

_______________

9. What is 'Bacteriology'?

_______________

10. What is it that is present in air and can be destroyed by heat?

_______________



## The Fight Against Infection

In 1796, Dr Edward Jenner inoculated a boy against the dreaded disease of smallpox which killed many thousands of people. He used a vaccine made from the cow-pox sores of a milkmaid. The boy caught the lesser disease of cow-pox and recovered but, when later inoculated with smallpox itself; he showed no signs of catching it. The practice of vaccination, as it came to be called, was quickly adopted throughout the western world. By 1801 at least one hundred thousand persons had been vaccinated in England.

When Pasteur carried out his researches on disease causing bacteria, he decided to adopt Jenner's idea of using a less deadly substance to vaccinate against a more dangerous disease. He found that some bacteria became inactive when cultivated outside the body, was able to produce vaccines from the inactive bacteria of a disease.

In the early 19th century many people were dying in hospitals from unknown causes when they should have recovered. Even minor operations proved fatal because the wounds became infected.

It was only after Pasteur had discovered that micro-organisms could be airborne, and proved that they caused infection, that hospitals and operating theatres were made cleaner. The man responsible for the greatest improvements in hospital conditions was a famous surgeon of the time, Joseph Lister. He invented a carbolic acid spray which was used in the operating theatre to kill bacteria in the air.

1. What did Dr Edward Jenner do in 1796?

   ______________________________

2. How many people were vaccinated in England?

   ______________________________

3. Bacteria become inactive when cultivated outside the body. Who said this?

   ______________________________

4. What was Louis Pasteur's research on?

   ______________________________

5. What happened in 19th century?

   ______________________________

6. What did Pasteur discovered?

   ______________________________

7. Who was Joseph Lister?

   ______________________________

8. What did he invent?

   ______________________________

9. Pasteur adopted ____________ idea in his researches on disease causing bacteria.

   (a) Joseph Listor's (b) Curie's (c) Jenncois (d) Newton's

10. 19th century saw unexplained deaths when patients were expected to recover. (True/False)

    ______________________________



## The Early Groping

The Age of the earth has been estimated to be about five billion years. Man is supposed to have arrived rather late in the earth's history—about a million years ago. We have recorded history of man only for the past 4000 to 5000 years. But if one goes through these records, however scanty they are, it is clear that man has always been at battle with his environment, with floods and drought, famine and warring neighbours. More than all these, mankind has been suffering from ravages brought about by pestilence and diseases. It was only a century ago that the enemy was identified and a systematic treatment of disease started; this is known Chemotherapy. It is essentially a contribution of the scientists of the 19th and 20th centuries. But it is impossible to visualize its full impact without understanding the historical perspective—the men and their fighting spirits through the ages which cumulatively helped in these discoveries.

1. What is the age of the earth estimated to be about?

   ______________________________

2. How old is man's arrival on earth?

   ______________________________

3. Man's history has been recorded for the past ____________ years.
4. In this record has man's life been uneventful?

   ______________________________

5. Name the events in the life of man as has been recorded

   ______________________________

6. __________ and ____________ have made mankind suffer huge losses.
7. Which treatment has been the gift of 19th and 20th century scientists?

   ______________________________

8. How does historical perspective help about the man involved in fighting diseases?

   ______________________________

9. When was the enemy of mankind identified?

   ______________________________

10. Fighting spirits through the ages have helped in the discovery of various treatment of diseases. (True/False)

    ______________________________

## Allergy to Penicillin

Very high levels of penicillin can be tolerated by man. There are, however, number of cases of allergic or hypersensitive reactions leading to death. According to recent concepts this sensitivity is caused by certain derivatives of penicillin associated with the pure molecule of penicillin. A skin test done with the penicillin to be injected to see hypersensitive reaction, if any, is a useful safeguard against such unfortunate fatalities.

### *Chloramphenicol (Chloromycetin)*

Chloramphenicol is effective against a wide range of organisms. It is active against a number of gram-negative and gram-positive bacteria and certain rickettsial infections. It is particularly useful in the treatment of typhoid fever caused by *Salmonella typhae* or *Salmonella paratyphi* A or B, infections which are notably resistant to all other antibiotics and chemotherapeutants.

1. Give the other name of Chloramphenicol.

 ______________________________

2. Chloramphenicol is useful against a wide ranged organisms. (True/False)

 ______________________________

3. What is it active against?

 ______________________________

4. Where is its particular use found in?

 ______________________________

5. Does *Salmonella paratyphi* A cause typhoid fever?

 ______________________________

6. How does *Salmonella typhae* become dangerous?

 ______________________________

## Whither Antibiotic Therapy?

The younger generation of people born the post-World War II era (after 1945) may not quite realize the magnitude of the problem faced by doctors when treating their parents and grandparents for infectious diseases before the advent of antibiotics. Today, thanks to the outstanding scientific contribution of the older generation, it is taken for granted that most disease-producing microbes can be eradicated by one drug or another. Before 1945, medical wards in hospitals always had a large number of young people seriously ill with diseases such as pneumonia, meningitis, septicaemia, while the post-operation wards were filled with patients having pus oozing out of abscesses, carbuncles and improper healing of surgical wounds. Now all this is changed due to the discovery of sulphanilamides, penicillin, streptomycin and a large array of antibiotics discovered in recent years. The advent of sulphanilamide drugs and antibiotics brought with it the promise that bacterial diseases might be brought under control, but that promise has not been fulfilled. Although many infections respond dramatically to chemotheraphy, tuberculosis, dysentery and typhoid fever continue to be endemic in many parts of the world, while cholera and plague erupt periodically; staphylococcal infection persists in the most advanced hospitals. One major reason for this is that the microorganisms have developed resistance to drugs.

When penicillin came on the scene it could easily eradicate staphylococci. However, by the mid-1950's as many as 90 percent of staphylococcal infections seen in hospital wards were associated with penicillin-resistant strains. Chloramphenicol and erythromycin were fortunately discovered in time to deal with the penicillin-resistant staphylococci and now, where strains resistant to all the three antibiotics are appearing, other synthetic derivatives of penicillin have been produced to deal with them.



## EXPRESSIONS USED TO DESCRIBE PERSON'S EXCITED FEELINGS

Many expressions may be used to describe someone who is excited.

### Beside Yourself

One such expression is to be "beside yourself." You can be beside yourself with anger or beside yourself with happiness, although usually not both at the same time. If you are beside yourself, you are in an extremely emotional condition. You are filled with excitement.

The dictionary tells us that "beside" means next to, or at the side of. So the expression "beside oneself" describes something that really not possible. You cannot be next to yourself. Some language experts, however, think the expression probably comes from an old belief that through magic, you could indeed be next to yourself. Spirits were believed to have the magic power to do anything. So it was possible to have two of the same person appear, especially if that person was excited.

Today, you might hear a husband say, "When my wife told me we were going to have a baby, I was beside myself with joy". Or someone might tell you he was beside himself with anger because he had lost his job.

When you are full of joy or are extremely excited about something you may do something else that is strange. You may "flip your lid". A lid is the cover that prevents something from escaping from a container. A lid on a cooking pot, for example, keeps the heat from escaping. To flip something is to turn it over. So, when you "flip your lid", you become so excited that your self-control escapes.

You can "flip your lid" over something you like very much. A young man, for example might flip his lid over a pretty, young woman. Or you can"flip your lid" if something makes you very angry. If some-one hits your new car it might make you flip your lid.

In recent years, the word "flip" itself has come to mean the same thing as flip your lid. It is common to hear a girl say she "flipped" over a new boyfriend.

An expression that means something quite similar is to "lose your head". The head is believed to be connected to reason and careful thought. Thus to "lose one's head" is to act without thinking, to be out of control.

1. What is the dictionary meaning of "beside"?

   ______________________________

2. "beside yourself" shows that you are in an extremely ____________ condition.

   ______________________________

3. How were spirits different from ordinary people?

   ______________________________

4. When was it possible to have two of the same person to appear?

   ______________________________

5. Give an example to show the emotional condition of a person in happiness.

   ______________________________

6. If the dictionary meaning is applied can the meaning be clear to the "husband-wife" situation shows here?

   ______________________________

7. Give reason for your answer.

_______________________________________________

8. Mention the strange thing done when one is filled with extreme excitement.

_______________________________________________

9. Why is the lid used on a cooking pot while cooking?

_______________________________________________

10. "Flip your lid actually" means .........

_______________________________________________

11. What is the modern equivalent of "Flip"?

_______________________________________________



## Black and White

Most of the time black and white appears as opposites. White means light and purity. Black is darkness and evil. But not always. Sometimes the words are used differently.

White hats and black hats represent the traditional meaning of the words. The hats are symbols of the "good guys" and the "bad guys" in American western movies.

White hats and black hats had a real purpose in the early days of motion pictures. The early movies were made with no sound. So, the movie directors put a white hat on the hero and a black hat on his opponent, the bad guy in the story. That way even a small child knew immediately who was the hero.

The tradition of white hats and black hats is no longer a part of movie making. But you still hear the expression when people talk about good guys and bad guys.

A "black sheep" is a person who does things that are not accepted, that violates tradition. A black sheep is rejected because he brings shame to his group. A family may have a member who is thought of as a black sheep, a person who is not welcome at family gatherings.

Black is also used in some expressions that describe good things. Being "in the black", for example, is a good situation for anyone. It is a business expression that means a company is earning money. A store that makes a profit is "in the black". The expression comes from the colour of the ink that is used in the books that record a company's profits or losses. Profits are written in black ink. Losses are written in red. So, when someone says his business is "in the red", he means it is losing money.

White usually means something good. A "white collar" job, for example, the kind of job many people seek. It is a job where you work at a desk, using your brain instead of your muscles. Usually white collar jobs pay more than "blue collar" jobs. Those are jobs where you use your muscles.

Sometimes white is used in an expression that is not good. Whitewash is such as expression. At first, whitewash meant to paint over something with a white paint to make it look better. But now "whitewash" has a different meaning: to hide or cover up mistakes or failures.

A newspaper might report, for example, the investigation of a train accident is a whitewash, because investigators did not really try to discover who was responsible.

Some expressions use black and white together. Someone may say to you that your proposal sounds all right, but he wants to see it in black and white. He wants to see your proposal in writing – black ink on white paper.

Some people are set to see things only in black and white. In this expression black and white represent opposite extremes with no middle ground between them. Most issues in the world are not so simple as black and white. One side of an issue is not all white – right or good – and the other side is not all black – wrong or evil. In the real world there are many grey areas where black and white mixed to represent the true situation.

1. How do Black and White generally appear as?

   ________________________________________________

2. What meanings are assigned to the two colours?

   ________________________________________________

3. Name the accessory that represents this traditional meaning.

   ________________________________________________

4. What do hats symbolise in western movies?

   ________________________________________________

5. When did the hats find a real purpose?

   ________________________________________________

6. How did the colours of hats matter in movies?

_______________________________________________

7. Who is a "blacksheep"?

_______________________________________________

8. How did small children know a hero and a villain?

_______________________________________________

9. Why is a person not welcome at family gatherings?

_______________________________________________

10. Profile are written in black ink. (True/False)

_______________________________________________



## Cross Your Fingers

The cross is an ancient symbol in many cultures and religions. It is closely linked, of course, with the Christian church. Scandinavian also used crosses to mark the edges of their territory. And the cross was sacred symbol to the Egyptians and to the Aztecs in Mexico. Today, the word across is used in many expressions that seem to have little direct connection to the religious beliefs.

For example, one way of wishing good luck to someone is to tell him that you will "keep your fingers crossed" for him.

Sometimes you may even cross two of your fingers when you wish him luck. But, more often, just saying the expression is believed to be enough to help bring success.

Crossing the fingers when making a wish may be tradition many hundreds of years old. But most experts think the expression in an American one that began about ninety years ago. It probably has its roots in the ancient Christian belief that making the sign of cross would keep away evil sprits and bad luck.

Children often cross their fingers when they tell a small lie. It is an old belief that lies will not be punished if told while the fingers are crossed. Many children have unhappily discovered that crossing their fingers offers no such protection.

Children often use another expression "cross my heart", when they say they are telling the truth. A child usually will make an X over his heart with his finger while saying it.

Language expert Charles Earle Funk says "cross my heart", and crossing the heart with the finger, probably come from the Roman Catholic Church tradition of making the sign of the cross. Mr. Funk also says that earlier in this century, children in the United States often expanded the simple saying. They said "Cross my heart and hope to die, and hope the cat will spit in your eye".

Cross is used in many other ways. If you deceive someone or confuse them you are "crossing them up".

And you might become "cross as two tricks" at someone. This old expression means you are very angry. What do two sticks have to do with the situation? If you put one stick across the middle of the other stick, you have a cross. And the word cross is another way to say angry. So if you are as cross as two sticks, then you are very angry.

Another expression, "to cross swords", sounds like something from the past. It recalls the period when knights in armor seemed to spend most of their time fighting. You can imagine two angry knights whose swords cross during a battle. But the expression no longer means a noisy fight with swords. It describes a less violent fight with words instead of swords. You "cross swords" with someone when you argue or debate an issue with him.

1. Cross is an ancient symbol in many cultures and religions. True or False?

______________________________________________________________________

2. Scandinavians use crosses to..........

3. What is the tradition behind people crossing their fingers?

______________________________________________________________________

4. Crossing the fingers has its root in the.......

5. What was the Christian belief of crossing the finger?

______________________________________________________________________

6. Why do children usually cross their fingers and what was the old belief of it?

______________________________________________________________________

7. What is the another most common expression used by the children and why do they use it?

______________________________________________________________________

8. What explanation did Charles Earle Funk give on the expression "cross my heart"?

______________________________________________________________________

9. What is the meaning of the expression " crossing them up", "cross as two tricks" and "to cross swords"?

____________________________________________

## Down-To-Earth, Both Feet on The Ground

"Down-to-earth" means being honest, open and easy to deal with.

It is a pleasure to find someone who is down-to-earth. A person who is down-to-earth is easy to talk to and accepts other people as equals. A down-to-earth person is someone who is opposite of someone who reacts to be important or proud.

Down-to-earth may be important members of the society, of course. But they do not let their importance "go to their heads". They do not consider themselves to be better than who are less important. Someone who is filled with his own importance and pride, often without cause, said to have "his nose in the air". There is no way a person with his nose in the air can be down-to-earth.

Americans use another expression similar to the ways to "down-to-earth". The expression is "both feet on the ground". Someone with both feet on the ground is a person with good understanding of reality. He has what is called "common sense".

He may have dreams, but he does not allow them to block his knowledge of what is real.

The opposite kind of person is one who has his "head in the clouds". A man with his head in the clouds is a dreamer whose mind is not in the real world.

Sometimes, such a dreamer can be brought back to reality. Sharp words from the teacher, for example, can usually get a day-dreaming student to put both feet back on the ground.

The person who is down-to-earth usually has both feet on the ground. But the opposite is not always true. Someone with both the feet on the ground may not be as open and easy to deal with as someone down-to-earth.

When we have both our feet firmly on the ground, when we are down-to-earth, we are realistic and we act honestly and openly toward others. Our lives are like the ground below us, solid and strong.

1. What is the meaning of the expression "Down-to-earth"?

____________________________________________

2. Who is a "Down-to-earth" person?

_______________________________________________

3. What does the expression "both feet on the ground" mean?

_______________________________________________

4. Opposite of the expression "both feet on the ground" is ........
5. Who is a man with his head in the clouds?

_______________________________________________

6. When we are down-to-earth, we are realistic. True of False?

_______________________________________________



## Go for It

The expressions "go for it"! is a way of urging someone to try something. "Go for it"! means you should not worry about failure, or be too careful. You should take a chance, be brave, and act firmly.

The expression comes from football. Not football as it is played in most countries, but the kind of football played in the United States and Canada.

American football is a difficult game to explain. But the basic idea is that each team tries to move the football across the goal line of the other team. A team must continue to move the ball steadily in the direction of the other team's goal line, or surrender it to the other team. One of the rules is that a term must move the ball ahead at least 10 yards—a little less than ten meters—in four attempts. It uses the ball to the other team if it fails to move that far.

One of the most exciting times in football comes when a team has failed, after three attempts, to move the ball forward ten yards. Then the team must make an important decision.

One choice is to try a fourth and final time to gain the remaining yards needed. If the team succeeds, it keeps the ball and continues to move forward. But if it fails, the other team gets the ball at that place on the field.

The second choice is to kick the ball. The team surrenders the ball if it makes this choice. But a good kick can put the other team at the far end of the field, making it more difficult for the team to score.

# Paragraph Writing

What should the team do? The conservative choice is to kick the ball. Accept temporary defeat to gain good position for the next time your team gets the ball. The more exciting choice, however, is to try a fourth and final time to gain the remaining yards needed.

People watching a football game are certain to shout their advice. Some will shout; "kick the ball!" but others will urge the team to take a choice, to live dangerously. "Go for it!" They will scream. "Go for it!"

In the 1980's people began using this expression in many kinds of situations to urge someone to take a chance.

For example, a student wants a date with the most beautiful student in his classroom. But he is not sure she will accept. "Go for it," His friends advice. "Ask her."

A young woman wants to buy an exciting dress. But it costs almost a week's pay. Should she buy it? "Go for it," her friends tell her. "Buy the dress."

There is no guarantee that the action you "go for" will succeed.

But that is the chance you take when you put your fears behind you and accept the unknown. You hold your breath, and you "go for it."

1. What is the meaning of the expression " Go for it"?

   ____________________________________________________________

2. From where does this expression come?

   ____________________________________________________________

3. How is football played?

   ____________________________________________________________

4. What is the rule that should be followed while playing football?

   ____________________________________________________________

5. What is the decision taken by the team when they fail?

   ____________________________________________________________

6. What are the reactions of the people when they watch the game?

   ____________________________________________________________

7. In what situations do we normally use this expression "go for it !"? Give examples.

________________________________________________

## Guinea Pig

Every language has its own special words and expressions. Often, they give new meaning to a common word or phrase. One such American expression is "guinea pig."

For centuries, scientists have used animals in medical experiments. They use animals to test new drugs and improve methods of operating on people.

One of the most commonly used animals in these experiments is the guinea pig. Someone hearing the name "guinea pig" for the first time might think this was a kind of pig that comes from the country of Guinea in West Africa. But the guinea pig is not part of the pig family. It looks more like a mouse or a rat. And the first guinea pigs came not from West Africa, but from South America, where they are called cavies.

The small long haired animals were raised by the Incas in Peru. They were first imported into Europe from South America in the 16th century. Some word experts say the word guinea in this case was a mistake in the way the word was spoken. They say the correct word was Guiana, a former British colony in South America now the country of Guyana. And they say it may have been called a pig because of the pig like, squealing sound it makes.

Scientists like to experiment on guinea pigs because the animals are small and are easy to control. They reproduce quickly and resist disease, making them valuable for laboratory tests. Scientists have used guinea pigs to test many important medicines.

For example, one of the most important medicines developed in recent years has been vaccine to control the chicken pox disease. Scientists in the United States tested the chicken pox vaccine on guinea pigs and other animals before testing it on humans.

Guinea pigs are not the only animals that scientists used in medical experiments. But they are among the most common. So, the expression, "guinea pigs" has come to mean more than just the name of the animals. Now, it means anything or anybody on which an experiment is done.

The army may choose a hundred soldiers as "guinea pigs" to test drive a new tank. Someone who likes to cook may invite some friends to dinner because she wants them to be "guinea pigs." She wants to know if her guests like the new kind food she has cooked.

# Paragraph Writing

The expression "guinea pig" probably is used more widely these days than real guinea pigs are used in medical experiments. Scientists have developed many experimental methods that allow them to do medical tests with a chemicals and computers instead of animals.

1. Why do scientists use animals in their medical experiments?

   ______________________________________________

2. Which is the most commonly used animal?

   ______________________________________________

3. Guinea pig belongs to the pig family. True of False?

   ______________________________________________

4. The first guinea pigs came from.........

5. What were they called as?

   ______________________________________________

6. What does the expression guinea pigs actually mean?

   ______________________________________________

7. Scientists have developed medical tests and chemicals in their experiments. True or False?

   ______________________________________________

## Rx

Some words and expressions are very old. Others have become part of our language only recently. The story goes back about 5000 years back.

It is about a sign that is used to represent some words.

We see the sign on drug stores and whenever we visit a doctor to get an order for medicine. It also appears on bottles of pills and other medicines.

The sign is formed by a line across the right foot of the letter "R". It represents the word "prescription." It has come to mean "take this medicine".

The sign has its beginnings 5000 years ago in Egypt. At the time, people prayed to Horus, the God of the Sun. It was said that when Horus was a child, he was attacked by Seth, the demon of evil.

The evil Seth put out the eye of the young Horus. The mother of Horus called for help. Her cry was answered by Thoth, the God of learning and magic. Thoth, with his wisdom and special powers, healed the eye of Horus, and the child was able to see again.

The ancient Egyptians used their drawing of the eye of Horus as a magic sign to protect themselves from disease, suffering and evil. They cut this sign in the stone they used for buildings. And it was painted on the papyrus rolls for writing about medicine and doctors.

For thousands of years, the eye of Horus remain as a sign of the God's help to the suffering and sick.

Long after the fall of the ancient Egyptian civilization, doctors and alchemists in Europe continued the custom of showing a sign of God's help and protection. But over the years, the sign changed from the eye of Horus to the sign for Jupiter, the chief God of Romans.

Jupiter sign looked much like the printed number "four."

That sign changed, also. Today it is the easily-recognized capital "R" with a line across its foot.

The sign no longer offers heavenly assistance to the sick. It now means "take this medicine."

Want more? Go ahead and read lots of books, magazines, newspapers, text-books and question your friends about all that you come across. Start a discussion. You have your question and answer exercises –verbally.

Now we come to the last aspect in reading skills.

1. How are words represented?

   ______________________________

2. How is the sign formed?

   ______________________________

3. Horus was .........and Seth was ........

   ______________________________

4. What did the Egyptians in their drawings use as a sign to protect themselves from diseases?

   ______________________________

5. The eye of Horus remained as..........for thousands of years.

   ______________________________

6. Why did the sign of the Eygptians change over years?

   ______________________________

7. What is the history behind the change of signs over the years?

______________________________________________

## Drawing Inference

Inference means the process of forming an opinion or finding out information indirectly based on what you already know.

You have to be careful; that you don't go overboard by your inferences—More than what is given.

Scanning helps in understanding BHTs, timetables, reading Index pages in books—this is found on the last page of every book. It helps in giving information quickly.

**I. Scan the railway time table given below and answer the given questions:**

| Bengaluru City | | | | | | |
|---|---|---|---|---|---|---|
| *Arrival from* | *Days for* | *Time* | *Departure* | *Time* | *Name* | *Days* |
| Ahmedabad | Thursday | 4:45 am | Ahmedabad | 13:30 hrs | Ahmedabad Express | Sunday |
| Chennai | Daily | 5:5 am | Chennai | 22:45 hrs | Blr-Chennai Mail | Daily |
| Mumbai | Sunday | 8:50 am | Mumbai | 20:15 hrs | Blr-Mumbai Express | Thu,Sun |
| Sholapur | Daily | 13:10 hrs | Yeshwanthpur | 14:10 hrs | 2628 | Daily |

i. Which train arrives on Sunday?

______________________________________________

ii. How many trains have their departure on Sundays from Bengaluru?

______________________________________________

iii. Do the trains arriving at Bengaluru city have names?

______________________________________________

iv. Does the train departing at 13:30 hours departure daily?

______________________________________________

v. If I need to go to South of India, which train do I take?

______________________________________________

vi. ____________________ trains arrive daily at Bengaluru city.

**II. You have a class-mate who is an enthusiastic sports fan. Help this person to write a time table to watch the relevant programme/s from 5 pm to 9 pm after scanning through these TV schedules.**

______________________________________________

______________________________________________

______________________________________________

______________________________________________

______________________________________________

______________________________________________

**III. You love to watch English movies. Here is the TV listing for Sunday. Scan and note down the details asked for:**

i. How many English movie channels do you recognize?

______________________________________________

ii. On which channel is Reporter's Diary?

______________________________________________

iii. If you have to watch the movie at 12:00 hrs and then another at 15:30 hrs, which channels need to be tuned into?

______________________________________________

iv. Which channel will air a serious movie at 23:00 hrs?

______________________________________________

v. How many channels have movie scheduled to start between 9:30 hrs and 10:30 hrs?

______________________________________________

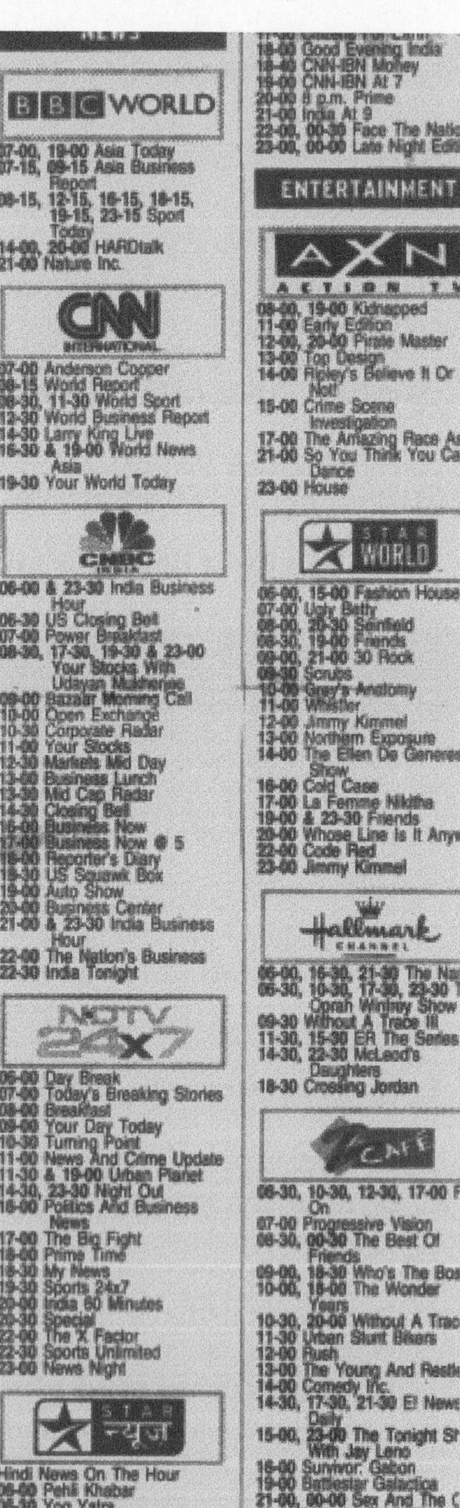

NEWS

BBC WORLD

07-00, 19-00 Asia Today
07-15, 09-15 Asia Business Report
08-15, 12-15, 16-15, 18-15, 19-15, 23-15 Sport Today
14-00, 20-00 HARDtalk
21-00 Nature Inc.

CNN INTERNATIONAL

07-00 Anderson Cooper
08-15 World Report
08-30, 11-30 World Sport
12-30 World Business Report
14-30 Larry King Live
16-30 & 19-00 World News Asia
19-30 Your World Today

CNBC INDIA

06-00 & 23-30 India Business Hour
06-30 US Closing Bell
07-00 Power Breakfast
08-30, 17-30, 19-30 & 23-00 Your Stocks With Udayan Mukherjee
09-00 Bazaar Morning Call
10-00 Open Exchange
10-30 Corporate Radar
11-00 Your Stocks
12-30 Markets Mid Day
13-00 Business Lunch
13-30 Mid Cap Radar
14-30 Closing Bell
16-00 Business Now
17-00 Business Now @ 5
18-00 Reporter's Diary
18-30 US Squawk Box
19-00 Auto Show
20-00 Business Center
21-00 & 23-30 India Business Hour
22-00 The Nation's Business
22-30 India Tonight

NDTV 24X7

06-00 Day Break
07-00 Today's Breaking Stories
08-00 Breakfast
09-00 Your Day Today
10-30 Turning Point
11-00 News And Crime Update
11-30 & 19-00 Urban Planet
14-30, 23-30 Night Out
16-00 Politics And Business News
17-00 The Big Fight
18-00 Prime Time
18-30 My News
19-30 Sports 24x7
20-00 India 60 Minutes
20-30 Special
22-00 The X Factor
22-30 Sports Unlimited
23-00 News Night

STAR न्यूज़

Hindi News On The Hour
06-00 Pehli Khabar
06-30 Yog Yatra
07-00, 09-30 Teen Deviyan
08-30 & 19-30 Wah Cricket

18-00 Good Evening India
18-40 CNN-IBN Money
19-00 CNN-IBN At 7
20-00 8 p.m. Prime
21-00 India At 9
22-00, 00-30 Face The Nation
23-00, 00-00 Late Night Editio

ENTERTAINMENT

AXN ACTION TV

08-00, 19-00 Kidnapped
11-00 Early Edition
12-00, 20-00 Pirate Master
13-00 Top Design
14-00 Ripley's Believe It Or Not!
15-00 Crime Scene Investigation
17-00 The Amazing Race Asi
21-00 So You Think You Can Dance
23-00 House

STAR WORLD

06-00, 15-00 Fashion House
07-00 Ugly Betty
08-00, 20-30 Seinfeld
08-30, 19-00 Friends
09-00, 21-00 30 Rock
09-30 Scrubs
10-00 Grey's Anatomy
11-00 Whistler
12-00 Jimmy Kimmel
13-00 Northern Exposure
14-00 The Ellen De Generes Show
16-00 Cold Case
17-00 La Femme Nikitha
19-00 & 23-30 Friends
20-00 Whose Line Is It Anyw
22-00 Code Red
23-00 Jimmy Kimmel

Hallmark CHANNEL

06-00, 16-30, 21-30 The Na
08-30, 10-30, 17-30, 23-30 T Oprah Winfrey Show
09-30 Without A Trace III
11-30, 15-30 ER The Series
14-30, 22-30 McLeod's Daughters
18-30 Crossing Jordan

CAFE

06-30, 10-30, 12-30, 17-00 F On
07-00 Progressive Vision
08-30, 00-30 The Best Of Friends
09-00, 18-30 Who's The Bos
10-00, 18-00 The Wonder Years
10-30, 20-00 Without A Trac
11-30 Urban Stunt Bikers
12-00 Rush
13-00 The Young And Restl
14-00 Comedy Inc.
14-30, 17-30, 21-30 E! News Daily
15-00, 23-00 The Tonight Sh With Jay Leno
16-00 Survivor: Gabon
19-00 Battlestar Galactica
21-00, 00-00 Sex And The C
22-00 I Wanna Be A Soap S

**IV. Here is an Index page from a reference book. Try to answer the points asked:**

**You find Index on the last page of every book. It helps in giving information quickly.**

| S. No. | Information | On Page |
|---|---|---|
| 1 | Perforated abdominal viscus | ________ |
| 2 | Lupus vulgaris | ________ |
| 3 | Mongolian blue spot | ________ |
| 4 | Silicon breast implants | ________ |
| 5 | Rickets | ________ |
| 6 | Kyphosis | ________ |
| 7 | Pulmonary embolism | ________ |
| 8 | Mucosal neuromas | ________ |
| 9 | Neurofibrosarcoma | ________ |
| 10 | Paget's disease (legs) | ________ |
| 11 | Ruptured biceps tendon | ________ |
| 12 | Superior vena cava obstruction | ________ |
| 13 | Ochronosis | ________ |
| 14 | Rheumatoid arthritis | ________ |
| 15 | Koilonychia | ________ |



i. How many entries have specifications given in the brackets?

______________________________________________

ii. There are __________ number of entries under N.

iii. Which are the entries given on two pages?

______________________________________________

iv. Which are the pages dealing with rheumatoid problems?

______________________________________________

v. Mention the hyphenated entries with page numbers.

______________________________________________

Here is a magazine Table of Contents.

January-March 2007 Volume 1 Number 1

## CONTENTS



**Answer the questions given below:**

1. What is the volume number?

___________________________________________

2. How many pages take up the topic Fetal Pleural Effusion?

___________________________________________

3. Give the library code given on this page.

___________________________________________

4. Who are the authors of Skeletal Anomalies?

5. On which page do you find polyhydramnios?

6. Themistoklis Mikos has written an article alongwith three others. True/False

7. Azen Salim is lone paper presenter on page 111. True/False

8. Prenatal Diagnosis is seen in three different paper presentations. Yes/No

9. If you want information on Conjoined Fetuses, which paper presentation would you turn to?

10. Who has authored the topic Nonimmune Hydrops Fetalis?

## Exercises

**I. Here is a conversation between two friends who meet at the mid-morning break. Read it quickly and see if you have understood it by answering the questions given:**

Nurse Radha : Hi Sam how is it in the wards?

Nurse Samantha : Hi and good night.

Nurse Radha : Oh! Oh! Poor you.

Nurse Samantha : Did you get the call from home?

Nurse Radha : Yes. My sister is coming over tomorrow.

Nurse Samantha : That's nice. What'll you do?

Nurse Radha : I have three tickets to see James Bond movie.

Nurse Samantha : Hmmm ....................

Nurse Radha : Do come. It'll be fun. After a long time ............. we can catch up.

Nurse Samantha : I have ER the whole day tomorrow.

1. Why does Nurse Samantha say good night?

______________________________________________

2. Is it really night?

______________________________________________

3. What does nurse Radha mean when she says poor you?

______________________________________________

4. Nurse Samantha's " hmmm-------" means she

______________________________________________

5. When Sam says she has ER the next day, what does she mean?

______________________________________________

**II. Read the telegram that Ruksana found among her grandfather's things when he asked her to clear his table.**

I Lost my purse—Stolen Send Rs 2000/—c/o Jug Lodge, 9th cross, David St, Colombo — Complaint given—Akbar.

Now let's see if you have enough inference.

1. Akbar is the name of her grand-father.

True/False

2. The sender doesn't have money.

   True/False

3. Is the person staying at Jug Lodge?

   ______________________________________________

4. What has Akbar done to get his purse back?

   ______________________________________________

5. Who is Akbar?

   ______________________________________________

**III. Here is an extract (a small piece from an article__extract) from a report given in the newspaper. Let's draw the inferences from it:**



Radha was at the nursing station at August Nursing Home. She was waiting to go off duty. Just at that moment a couple walked into the hospital. They were directed to meet nurse Radha. She quickly understood that the man required medical assistance. She quickly asked questions. She found that a continued stomach pain along with vomiting five times had brought the couple to the hospital. She continued to ask questions and started recording the man's answers. Occassionally, the wife would add points. She took his temperature which was normal. The Spyhgmomagnometer gave his blood pressure to be slightly high. His pulse rate was recorded. She then checked his weight and height. For a slim man he weighed 70 kgs, When he stood on the weighting machine, the complained of ringing in the ears. When asked the man told his name to be Sandesh Bhat. Mrs Sharada Bhat told the nurse that he had a past history of ear infection, but the ENT Surgeon Dr Ali Khan had helped in curing it. To meet Dr Ali they had travelled to Hyderabad by plane a few years earlier. Mrs Bhat softly added that the problem begun after Mr Bhat had later some Thai food which he was not used to. The various instruments in the nursing station made Mr Bhat wish to just go away from all these white-coated people. He looked gloomy. Nurse Radha recorded all this and now she felt she could send them to Dr Solomon with the details she had recorded. By this time nurse Edwina came to relieve nurse Radha. She waited for Radha to come out of the consultation room. Before Radha left for home, she briefed nurse Edwina about the work and the patient who had come in.

1. ______________________________________________
______________________________________________
2. ______________________________________________
______________________________________________
3. ______________________________________________
______________________________________________
4. ______________________________________________
______________________________________________
5. ______________________________________________
______________________________________________
6. ______________________________________________

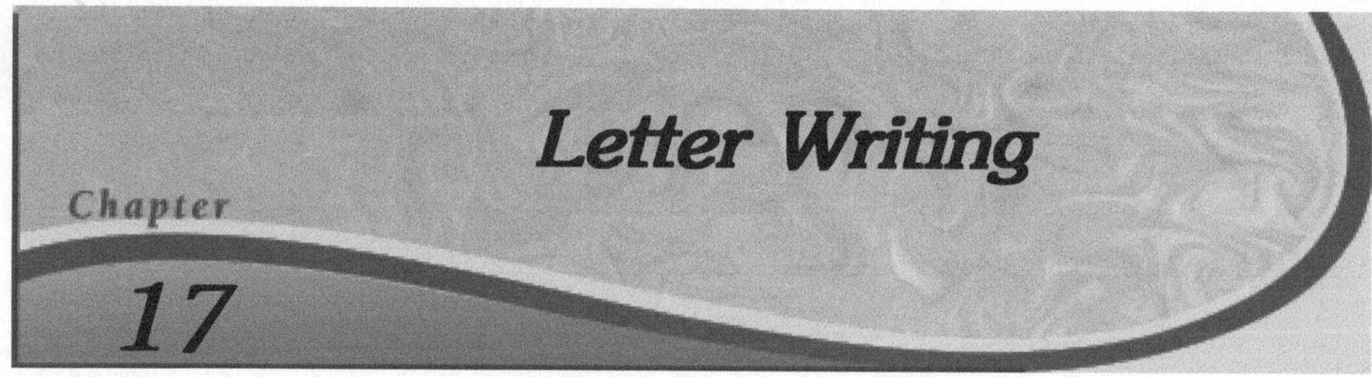

# Chapter 17 Letter Writing

Look at these:

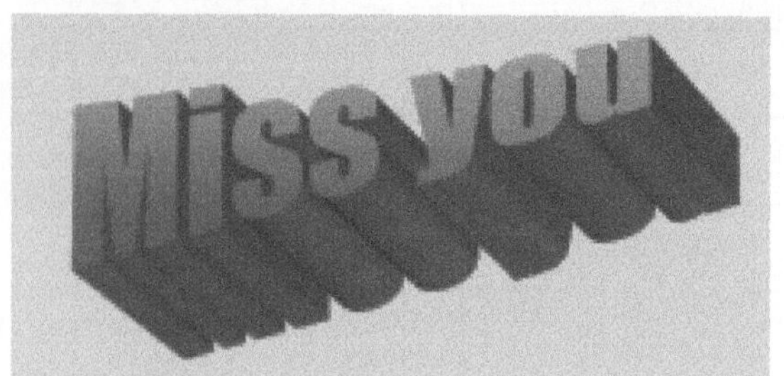


Hi Mom,
I've gone to Joji's place. 'll be back by dinner time.
The cat has had the bath.
♥
Ajay

Cinema tickets are with Rocky
C u
Later alligator.

In our lives we write letters to various people for various reasons. In today's world, when e-mail has taken over the communication routes along with the mobile phones, many people feel that writing letters has become obsolete. But don't you remember the small note which you wrote saying 'thank you' and left it on the fridge or table or pinned on the pillow? Or the small individual messages which are shown above?

Even that note is letter writing. The human mind always feels secure when it sees a written communication. Some years ago writing letters was the cheapest means of communication. Today it is called 'snail mail'. This is because quicker communications like e-mail, SMSs are available. Even the letters sent by e-mail require some knowledge of writing letters. All through our lives, we do write letters for different reasons. Thus, we need to look at some guidelines for writing a properly worded letter.

Today, though we use e-mail and mobile for quick communication, we need to write different kinds of letter to different people for various reasons. For example, we need to write letters of applications to join university courses or request information about a particular course or write to our friends. Apart from this, we may need to write letters to officials in an organization or to the officials in the government or to newspapers for various reasons. Therefore, it is vital to know how to write letters.

There are two kinds of letters.

1. Formal letters or non- personal letters.
2. Informal letters or personal letters.

# Letter Writing

**Formal Letters:** These are letters written for business purposes.

**Informal Letters:** These are letters written to close relatives and friends.

Each letter has its own particular form; but there are certain points which apply to all. Let us take up the two kinds, one by one.

Let us first take the layout of a formal letter or a non-personal letter.

|  |  |
|---|---|
| 97/2, 8th Cross, 3rd Main<br>Crescent Street<br>Bengaluru-560045 | Sender's address (From) |
| 3 January 2009 | Date |
| Anand Khan<br>Consultant<br>Mary Radiology Centre<br>Vellore. | Receiver's address (To) |
| Dear Mr Khan, | Salutation |
| ____________________ | Body of letter |
| With regards<br>Yours sincerely | Complimentary closes |
| *anita Rodrigues* | **signature** |
| Anita Rodrigues | Name typed |
| Staff Nurse | Title or Position |
| Enc encloses. | |

Chapter 17

In this layout we observe that From, To and punctuation marks like commas and fullstops have been omitted. When you write the letter, you add the punctuation marks.

Now let us take each feature and understand the role it plays.

***Sender's address or 'From' address:*** The first entry in a letter is on the left hand side close to the margin of the page. It may or may not include the name.

***Date*** The second entry in a letter is on the left hand side below the address. The separation is a space between the sender's address and date. The 'th' in the date is dropped these days (4th). To avoid confusion, better write the month in words. For example, 02.03.2008 in United Kingdom means 2$^{nd}$ of March 2008. But in the US it means February 3rd 2008.

***Receiver's address or 'To' address:*** The third entry in a letter is on the left hand side below the date. It includes the receiver's name, title and address. If the name of the person is not known, the person's (his or her) title or designation in the institution or company is written. (like The Director, The Matron, The Principal).



One can also address a letter to a particular department in the institution or company.

If a situation arises where one does not know anything about the person (i.e., his/her name, title) or about the institution or company and one does not want to assume anything, the letter should be addressed to the institution or the company itself.

***Punctuation:*** When punctuation is used in the address, each line of the address is followed by a comma, except the last line. These days, there is a tendency to write letters without any commas as shown.

***Salutations:*** This means the words that are used in a letter to address the person one is writing to. The word salutation also means something that you say to welcome or greet somebody; the action of welcoming or saying hello to somebody is called salutation.

***For example:*** Dear Sir, Respected Sir/Madam (This is not in frequent use now).

There are a few points one needs to keep in mind while using salutations.

They are:

i. The first name of the person is used only when he/she is well-known to the person writing the letter.

ii. Use the person's surname if you know it. (Like Dear Mr. Rathode or Dear Miss Rao.)

iii. Dear Sir is to be used when you are writing to a man and don't know his name.

iv. Dear Madam is to be used when you are writing to a woman and don't know her name.

v. Dear Sir/Madam is to be used when you are writing a letter without knowing the gender or name of the person you are writing to.

(Ex: Editor of a newspaper, principal of an institution which you are applying for or a doctor, etc. These days you have both men and women in every position in the professional field).

You can also do away with Sir/Madam and replace it with the position the person holds like Dear Editor, Dear Principal, and so on. In some countries Respected is preferred in place of Dear.

## *Complimentary Closes*

When you finish writing the letters, you have to close the letter. You can write Best wishes, Regards, Warm regards, etc. in letters which are not very formal and if you know the person or have spoken to them often on the phone.

***Note # 1:*** You have to use Yours faithfully if you have used Dear Sir or Dear Madam in the salutation of your letter.

***Note # 2:*** You have to use Yours sincerely if you have used the person's name in the salutations (Like Dear Mr. Joseph or Dear Lovella).

### *Body of the Letter*

As a letter is a written piece of communication, the content should be brief, complete and, above all, relevant to the purpose for which it is written. This is in case of a formal letter which may be a letter seeking or giving information on a particular topic or event. In case of an informal letter you can write as many details you want the receiver to know.

Let's take the formal letter. If you are writing a letter seeking or giving information or writing a letter of complaint, divide the letter into three parts so that you can be better organized and coherent. This will help you in remembering all the points to be included in the letter.

The three divisions are:

- Introduction which tells who you are and the reason you are writing the letter.
- The actual reason which shows whether you are seeking or giving information.
- Conclusion which tells what is expected from the receiver.

***Signature, Name typed, Title or Position:***

When the letter that you are writing is a formal one, then the need of your name typed below the signature is needed along with the title or position.

If you are writing an informal letter, then your signature would be known to the person and your title and designation would be ludicrous.

***Enclosures:***

These are required only when you write formal letters.

Now here are two letters, identify the types they belong to

Rose Cottage
Allahabad, 12,
2nd December 19 – –

Dear John,
Can you guess what I did yesterday? I had my first ride in a motor car! Shri. Dinanath, who is a friend of father, brought his car round yesterday afternoon, and took us all for a drive.

I mean to have a car and drive it myself when I grow up. So what if I am a girl? Nobody's clothes got dirty. It was such a relief to be in a vehicle that takes care of all the minute important things.

Well, I must stop. Good-bye!

With love from
Henry

14, Temple St.
Mysore 23.
8th April 2007

The Director,
Indus
No. 19, RV Road,
Bengaluru 4.

Dear Sir,
I saw your advertisement for CAT coaching classes in Times of India dated 4th April 2007. Could you please send me a copy of your brochure and details of payment, classes and last date for joining?

Thank you,
Your faithfully
Narain

**1. This is a ____________________ letter.**
**2. This is a ____________________ letter.**

## Exercises

**I. Now looking at the formal letter put the following in the correct orders (You can use nos 1-10 or 1st, 2nd so on).**

__________________Name typed

__________________Enclosures

__________________Salutation

__________________Signature

__________________Sender's address

__________________Title or Position

____________________ Receiver's address

____________________ Complimentary close

____________________ Date

____________________ Body of the letter

**Now look at the informal letter and tell the order of the parts of the letter. (Use numbers like the previous ones).**

____________________ Body of the letter

____________________ Signature

____________________ Date

____________________ Sender's address

____________________ Salutation

____________________ Complimentary closes.



**II. Here is a letter written by a student nurse to the principal seeking permission to attend a workshop on presentation skills. Identify the mistakes, put the points in the correct order and rewrite the letter.**

> Dear Sir,
>
> Although I have been chosen to attend the workshop, I need to go to the Chennai for this College and practical classes going is on now and I have left this.
>
> My presentation skills is not up to mark. So, I have to go myself learning better methods. So, I wanting to permission for go you.
>
> You will kindly requesting your goodself to grant 1 week leave September 9th starting 7 days. The letter from workshop organizers are here.
>
> Your's warm regards
>
> Sincerely
>
> Sudha a costa

Now re-write the letter in the space provided.

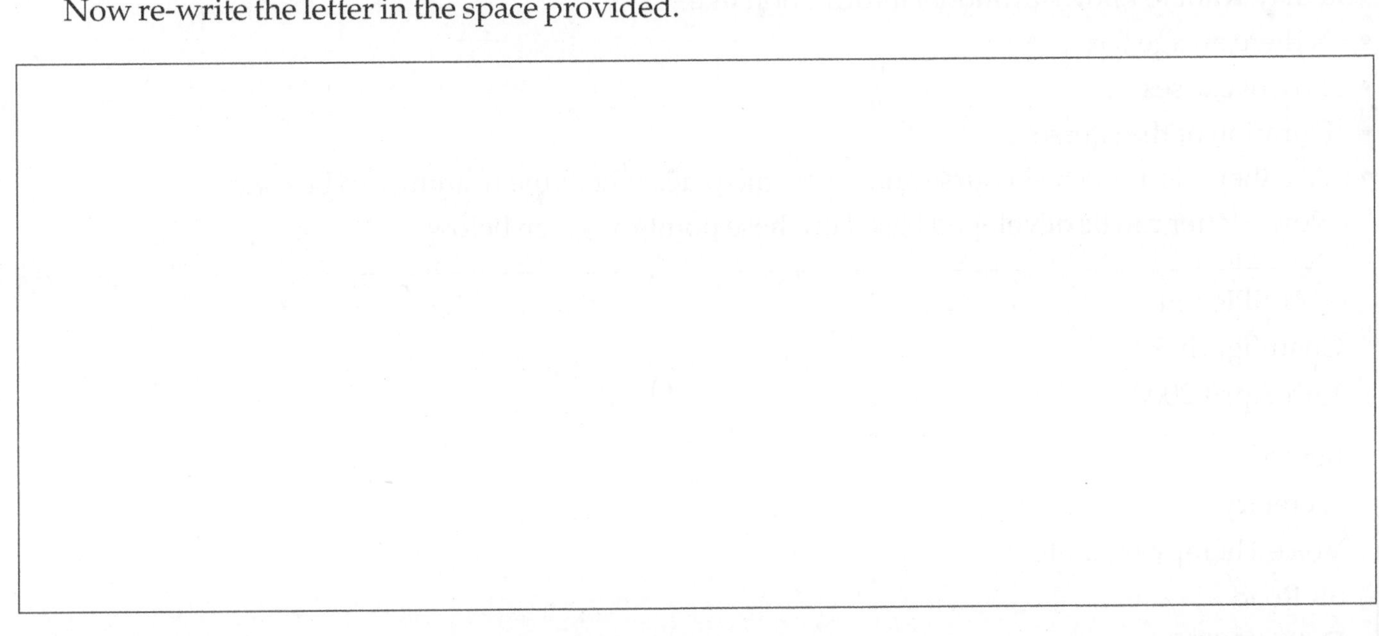

To learn letter writing in an easy method we shall divide the types of letters according to our needs. This is not a complete list. You as the learner must remember that there are different types of letters in different professions in this world. Here we will deal with those letters that help us in a general way as well as in a specific context.

## Letter Seeking Information or Permission

Everyday you notice the advertisements given in a newspaper. It may be for finding a reasonably good priced house to rent, a second hand vehicle to buy, a college to seek admission or many are the times you will be looking at the possibilities of various jobs and vacancies in there for yourself. When you come across something that suits you, you write a letter or go along letters are called as letters seeking information.

You see the following advertisement in a newspaper.

Voice training will be given.
Classes begin on March 9th
For details contact: Revoli
Secretary, Voice Therapy Institute
SR Road, Delhi 110017.

You may want to know additional information like–

- Is there an age bar
- Cost of classes
- Duration of the course
- Whether it is a certified course and if yes, the place where the training can be used.

Now a letter can be developed based on these points as given below.

38/1 SPRV St.,
Chandigarh 5
19th April 2008

Revoli
Secretary
Voice Therapy Institute
SR Road
Delhi 110017.

Dear Mr Revoli

I am a student nurse. I am studying in my second year. I read the advertisement on the voice training classes in the newspaper Times of India dated 17th April 2008. Would you please send me a copy of your brochure and include information as to whether it is a certified course and places. I would also like to know if there is an age bar to take up these classes. What would be the cost and duration of the course?

Please send me an application form also.
Thank you
Yours sincerely

(Joseph A Reed)

## Exercise

1. Samuel Emanuel is in his last year of undergraduate studies in nursing. He wants to continue his studies by taking up Masters Programme in Nursing and Management. Write a letter to the Director of the institution which has such a programme. Your letter must contain–

- Duration of course
- Course fee
- Enquiry if job placements are taken care of by the institution
- Hospital work that is expected in the course.

2. Your class wants to go on a week long tour to a sea-side resort before the final year classes are closed. As the class leader, write a letter to a tourist bureau seeking information for an affordable place to go. Your letter should contain–
   - Group travel discount and student discount
   - No. of places you can visit
   - Accommodation details
   - Food for all–vegetarian and non-vegetarian.



## Leave Letters (Letters Seeking Permission)

You need to go home as your parents need your help for a few days. This is due to fractures your parents sustained due to an accident. Write a letter requesting your Principal to grant you leave of absence from your classes for two weeks.

-------------------------

1st year BSc Nursing

3rd February 2009

Principal

Altazar Nursing College

Dear Sir,

My parents have sustained fractures in an accident recently in my home town. I received this information just a few minutes before. I need to be home to look after them.

Kindly give me permission to go home for two weeks and help my parents in their hour of need. I promise to keep up my studies and not to allow this absence of two weeks from my classes to affect my academics.

Your obedient student

-------------------------

## Exercise

1. Write a leave letter to the head of your department to give you permission to submit your records three weeks later as you are going home to take care of your parents.
2. Write a leave letter addressed to the head of your department requesting permission not to attend to your duties in the hospital as you have viral fever.

## Letters Giving Information

Sometimes you will be in a situation where you are asked to give information sought by people who are unknown to you or, as part of your duties you are expected to write letters giving the information asked for. Such letters are called as letters giving information.

Imagine you are the student vice-president of the college. Your college is conducting a competition for nursing students in debate and essay writing. You need to draft a letter giving details of this programme to the Principals of all nursing colleges in your district/city.

When you compose such a letter, you need to remember certain points like–

- A sentence or two about your college.
- Details about the debate and essay writing competitions—It is a regular affair or done for first time.
- Facilities provided/participation fee/eligibility/number of prizes/how to apply.
- Last date for entries/On-spot entry.
- When the topics will be given.

*Note:*

1. If a letter like this is written on the college letter head the 'From Address' is not required. But in an exam and to practise, you are expected to write the 'From Address'.
2. As the letter drafted is common to all colleges, the names of the heads of the various institutions need not be written.
3. Sir/Madam should be written as the post of a Principal can be held by a man or a woman.

9th January 2009

Dear Sir/Madam,

St. Clare Nursing College is a twenty-year-old institution upholding the guidelines put forth by Florence Nightingale for nurses.

Every year it is a tradition to hold inter-collegiate competitions on the Foundation Day. This is by invitation only. The competition is organized for first and second year nursing under-graduate students. This is held on 2nd February. I wish to invite your college students to participate in this competition and exhibit their skills in public speaking and writing.

The competitions are Debate and Essay writing in English. The college has instituted three prizes in each competition for the deserving students. The debate will be held in the college auditorium and will begin at 10 am sharp. Mike will be provided to the participants. Each speaker has 4 minutes to speak. Only two participants per college are allowed in debate. One must talk **for** the given topic and the other must talk **against** the given topic.

The essay writing competition will be held on the same day in the classrooms G-1 and G-2. Writing paper and pen will be provided to all participants. Only one student per college is eligible to participate in this competition.

There is an entry fee of Rs. 25 per participant, be it debate or essay writing. Depending on the situation on-the-spot entries will be allowed. Participants should fill in the enclosed entry forms.

The topics will be told telephonically two days prior to the competition. Kindly send in the complete entry form by the 20th of January 2009.

Thank you
Yours faithfully,

*Archana Raghavendra*
Vice-President

Enc. Entry form

## Exercise

You are given the duty to be a student counsellor. You have to draft a letter to a prospective nursing student Miss Charlotte Gonzalvance giving her the information about your college. Your letter must include the activities conducted in your college, the curriculum she can expect and the college timings.

Finally, you come to the section which all of you must learn in order to get ahead in your professional lives. Once the under-graduate or post-graduate study is over, to get a job, one must apply for the posts available. This requires what we call CV-Curriculum Vitae attached to a formal letter. How should such a letter be drafted or composed? Here is an example.

### Curriculum Vitae

**Name in full** : Rajatha Fernandes

**Date of birth** : 18.06.1973

**Address** : 276, 8th Cross, 7th Main Road,
III Stage, Frazer Town,
Bengaluru

**Telephone No.** : 080-63425845

**Educational Qualifications:**

| Sl. No. | Institution Attended | Year | Course | Grade |
|---|---|---|---|---|
| 1 | RSVE School, Bengaluru | 1988 | 10th Standard/SSLC | First Class |
| 2 | ST. Augustine PU College, Goa | 1990 | 12th Standard/PUC | First Class |
| 3 | JV Nursing College, Mangalore | 1994 | BSc Nursing | First Class |
| 4 | St. Alameda, Delhi | 1996 | MSc Nursing | First Class |

**Work Experience:** Worked for two years as a junior nurse in Government Hospital, Delhi from 1996-1998.

Worked in Radiology Department for three years in Anand Hospital from 1999-2001.

Currently working as a senior nurse in the Casualty Department at Apollo Glow Group of Hospitals, Bengaluru.

**Salary drawn** : Rs. 12000 per month.

**References:**

1. Head Nurse at Government Hospital, Delhi
2. Head Radiology Anand Hospital.
3. Head Casualty Department Apollo Glow Group of Hospitals, Bengaluru.
4. Testimonial from the Principal St. Alameda's, Delhi.

Now this CV must be attached to a formal Letter of Application as shown.

Rajatha Fernandes
276, 8th Cross, 7th Main Road,
III Stage, Frazer Town, Bengaluru

16.02.2008

Director,
Mani Group of Hospitals,
Mangalore.

Dear Sir/Madam,

My name is Rajatha Fernandes working in Apollo Glow Group of Hospitals in Bengaluru. I read your advertisement for Head Nurse in Casualty Department in the Deccan Herald newspaper dated 2nd February 2008.

I am interested to work in your esteemed organization. I feel I can take this responsible task as I have the necessary experience and qualification. I have enclosed my CV and reference letters. If any clarification is required, I will be glad to provide it.

Hope to hear a positive response from you.

Thank you
Yours faithfully

*Rajatha Fernandes*

(Rajatha Fernandes)
Encl. 1. CV
2. Reference letters

## Exercise

1. Now try to draft your CV and application letter.
2. Given a newspaper advertisement. Write a letter answering this.

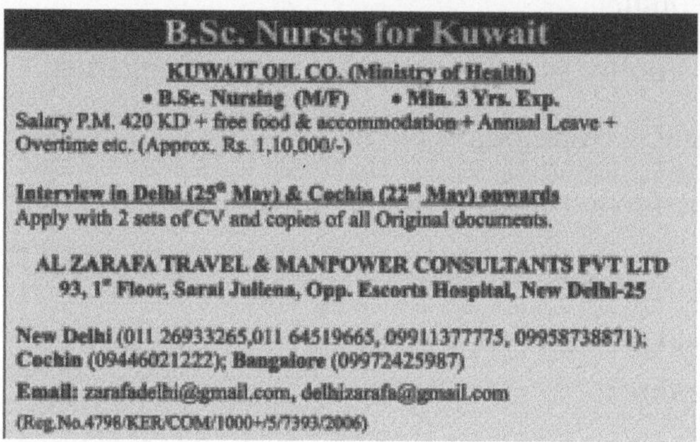


This completes your training in this section. Let us now move to the next interesting section.

# Part IV

- All About Using a Dictionary
- Report Writing

Chapter 18

# All About Using a Dictionary

Many are the times we come across words which we do not know. Many are the times we know the words yet we cannot recall the meaning of the word. Sometimes, we are stunned when the word we know is used by somebody to give a different meaning. These are the times we use a book that helps us in giving all the required information. This book contains all the words in the English language and it only shows the different meanings but how one uses the word just in a sentence. This book gives the information about the word—the part of speech it belongs to. This book is the dictionary.

Here, we learn more about the dictionary and the work it does in our lives. No student can afford to say "I don't need a dictionary."

One must never get to put off by the sheer size of the dictionary. Once one learns how to use this wonderful book, it is sheer pleasure to use it and to read it. Yes! Read it! After all it is a book too.

When one opens a dictionary the first few pages give a lot of information. This information helps a person in using the dictionary. Let us get acquainted in using a dictionary.

The first information we get is a page titled ABBREVIATIONS. Abbreviations mean short form of a word or phrase. These days people are busy forming short forms of messages to save space while using SMS in a mobile. Each person creates his/her own version of a short form of a word or phrase. Here are the standard short forms. These are common in all the dictionaries.

*For example:* abbr- abbreviation
Adj- adjective
Sb- somebody

The list is long. These abbreviated forms help in printing all the information about the word in a dictionary.

## Exercise

Look up the list of abbreviation in a dictionary and write the complete forms of the given abbreviations:

1. Adv ____________________
2. App ____________________
3. Arch____________________
4. Art ____________________
5. Aux ____________________
6. Brit ____________________
7. Conj ____________________
8. Comb form ______________
9. Def ____________________
10. Derog __________________
11. Esp____________________
12. Euph __________________
13. Fem ____________________
14. Fig ____________________
15. Fml ____________________
16. Idm ____________________
17. Joc ____________________
18. N ______________________
19. Pl ______________________
20. Pp _____________________
21. Illus ____________________
22. Pt ______________________
23. Sing ____________________
24. Sl ______________________
25. Sth _____________________

26. Symb ____________________

27. Us ____________________

28. Usu ____________________

29. V ____________________

30. Sr. No. ____________________

Some dictionaries give this on the backside of the face cover, some give this on a separate sheet.

Next we come across the Phonetic Symbols. These show how a word should be pronounced. Both the vowel and consonant sounds are given. It looks like this:

1. i
2. I
3. e
4. æ
5. a: and so on

These symbols are given along with the words showing the sound that is produced by them. For example,

I. i: as in see/si:/

That is, i: whenever one sees this symbol one must pronounce see sound.

II. æ Yes, this looks like 'a' and 'e' are sticking together. When one comes across this symbol, one must produce the 'a' sound as in 'hat'

That is, æ as in hat/hæt/

After Phonetic Symbols, we get 'Key to Entries' or how to understand the printed matter in a dictionary. Let us take the word 'lime'. This is how the dictionary entry is.

Lime'/I aim/ n [U] 1 (also ' quicklime) white
Substance (Calcium oxide) obtained by heating
Limestone, used in making cement and mortar
And as a fertilizer. 2 = BIRDLIME (BIRD)

***Extra matter***

pronunciation of the head word.

Number of the definitions

Different word used with the same meaning.

Definition/meaning of the head word.

Grammatical information about nouns

Part of speech.

Let us take another word anaemia. In a dictionary the word and the associated information is printed in the following manner.

an. ae.mia Us ane.mia/ a'ni:mia n [U] (medical)

Condition of the blood caused by a lack of red corpuscles, making the person look pale.



***Extra matter***

Head word

Pronunciation of the head word with the different spellings/pronunciations used by speakers of American English

Part of speech grammatical info about nouns.

an.aemic (US an.emic) a'ni:mik/adj

Numbe of the definition

Suffering from or showing the symptoms of anaemia: She looks anaemic in my opinion.

Now we come to learn how to find the word we want in any standard dictionary. There are certain steps followed in finding the word and the information associated with it.

For ease of learning, consider the word **'Context'**. The given word starts with 'C' so, first open the 'C' section in the dictionary.

You would feel tense or apprehensive as there are many words under 'C'. Don't get tense or irritated. Initially, it takes some time and patience to learn how to find a word. Once you learn, it becomes very easy.

The second step is to consider the first and second letters of the word given. Here it is 'Co' [keep open the pages under the alphabet 'c']. You would have noticed that every page in a dictionary has two words printed at the top.

**Con-text**/'kontekst/*n*[C, U] 1 Words that come before and after a word, phrase, statement, etc. helping to show what its meaning is: *Can't you guess the meaning of the word from the context? O Don't quote my words out of context*, e.g. so as to mislead people about what I mean. 2 circumstances in which sth happens or in which sth is to be considered: In the context of the present economic crisis it seems unwise to lower taxes. *O you have to see these changes in context: they're part of a larger plan.*

**Con-tex.tual**/kan'tekstsval/adj of or according to context: Contextual clues can help one to find the meaning.

Look at these words as you turn the pages. Initially, you get the words starting with the letter ca' then words starting with the letters 'ca' and 'ce' on the some page. As you keep turning the pages, you finally get page where the words begin with the letter 'Co'. Here again you have a huge list . Now take the third and fourth letter along with the first two. That is, you now check the/1st beginning with 'cont'. You will get a comparatively smaller list. Yet, you immediately don't get the word context. You see words starting with 'conta'. So, you will 've to consider the 5th letter 'e'. Therefore you have conte. You get the pages with head words container and content' then the page with the head words 'contention and continue'. You now realize the word you are searching for is on the page that has the head word 'contention and continue'. This is because the word we are searching for lies somewhere between these two head-words. So we keep our finger on the head words and go down the page, and we come across the word we are looking for context. Look at the box showing the dictionary entry with the said head words.

This is the process of looking-up a word in any dictionary.

Now let us look at the entry for context and understand the information give in a dictionary. Let us apply all that we have learnt here.

First we see that the above word is a noun. It can be used both as a countable noun and as an uncountable noun.

Second we see that it has two different meanings in usage. Third point we notice is that there is an adjectival form too.

So the three different sentences given here are:

1. Can't you guess the meaning of the word from the context?
2. In the context of the present economic c crisis it seems unwise to lower taxes.
3. Contextual clues can help one to find the meaning.
1. Helps us to understand the meaning of a word with respect to something.
2. The circumstance in which taxes cannot be reduced.
3. Gives the adjectival usage. This sentence that a certain situation or picture given helps in understanding a word.

There are many words in a dictionary that have more than three meanings. Reading a dictionary or looking-up words in a dictionary helps us to know the different ways in which we have to use a word.

Now let as apply all that we have learnt about how to use dictionary in doing the exercises given below.



## Exercise

Some words are given below. Find the Parts of Speech they belong to from a dictionary. Note a few may have more than one form.

| | |
|---|---|
| 1. above——————— | 6. fasten ——————— |
| 2. blow——————— | 7. gag ——————— |
| 3. cash——————— | 8. here ——————— |
| 4. deaf——————— | 9. I ——————— |
| 5. elated——————— | 10. Jack-daw ——————— |

Are you now clear about this aspect with a word? If yes let's move on. If not I would suggest you ask your friends to give you some more words so you can practice some more and understand the process.

Here are some words. Write the different definitions or meanings associated with them. Use a dictionary to do this.

1. hunt

2. instruct

3. lead

4. logic

5. old

Now use the same head words and form sentences of your own giving the different meanings in the space provided.

1. ______
2. ______
3. ______
4. ______
5. ______
6. ______
7. ______
8. ______
9. ______
10. ______
11. ______
12. ______
13. ______
14. ______
15. ______
16. ______
17. ______
18. ______
19. ______
20. ______
21. ______
22. ______
23. ______

24. ____________________

25. ____________________

26. ____________________

By now you will have realized that you are able to comprehend and construct sentences using the same word in giving different meanings.

## Tip

Read as many books both fictions and non-fiction to see the way words are used thus expanding your vocabulary, knowledge and your ability to crack jokes by playing with words.

When we talk about words, you would have noticed certain words as you turned the pages of a dictionary. They would have intrigued you. (don't know the meaning of 'intrigue' ? The dictionary is in front of you ☺) Let us now know a bit more about these words.

There is no classification of words other than putting them under parts of speech. But, to understand the various uses of a word and for ease of learning here is a short classification or types of words. Mind you, all the words in the English language cannot be put under these types. This classification is to draw your attention to the interesting aspect of the language.

You remember we come across compound words in the chapter Nouns?

Let me refresh your memory.

*Compound word:* Two or more different words put together to form a word that gives a different meaning from the root words.

Ex: Grand and father → grand-father

Son and in and law → Son-in-law.

You find a lot of compound words in the dictionary.

Write 15 compound words in the dictionary.

1. ____________________
2. ____________________
3. ____________________

4. ______________________________

5. ______________________________

6. ______________________________

7. ______________________________

8. ______________________________

9. ______________________________

10. ______________________________

11. ______________________________

12. ______________________________

13. ______________________________

14. ______________________________

15. ______________________________



**Synonyms:** Words giving meanings that are similar.

Ex: *Slay, Kill*

These two words mean to finish off a person or take-away the life of a person.

**Antonyms:** Words which give the opposite meanings of the given word.

Ex: *Fast* and *slow*

*Young* and *old*

**Homonyms:** Words that are spelt and pronounced a similar way but the meanings differ.

Ex: *Miss*

1. an unmarried lady.
2. a school teacher is addressed by her students with this.
3. fail to catch, hit or reach something

**Homophones:** Words that are different and have different meanings but sound the same.

Ex: board → long thin flat piece of cut wood used for building walls, boats, etc.

bored → feeling uninterested.

## Exercises

**I. Give the Antonyms of following words.**

| | | | | | |
|---|---|---|---|---|---|
| Progress | ____________ | Smart | ____________ | Calm | ____________ |
| Cold | ____________ | Night | ____________ | Can | ____________ |
| Warm | ____________ | Huge | ____________ | Finite | ____________ |
| Intelligent | ____________ | Slim | ____________ | Build | ____________ |
| Sweet | ____________ | Open | ____________ | Strict | ____________ |

**II. Give the meanings of these Homonyms**

1. Match ________________________________________
2. Race ________________________________________
3. Board ________________________________________
4. Present ________________________________________
5. Pitcher ________________________________________
6. Card ________________________________________

**III. Give the Synonyms of:**

1. Hop ____________________
2. Home ____________________
3. Content ____________________
4. Lonely ____________________
5. Fast ____________________
6. Same ____________________
7. Various ____________________
8. Build ____________________
9. Sever ____________________
10. Wither ____________________

**IV. Give the Homophones of the following words:**

1. Knew ____________________
2. No ____________________
3. Rain ____________________
4. Whether ____________________
5. Fair ____________________
6. Pale ____________________
7. Fare ____________________
8. Right ____________________
9. Weight ____________________
10. Peace ____________________
11. Been ____________________
12. Dew ____________________
13. Check ____________________
14. By ____________________
15. Pain ____________________

With this we come to the end of the interesting chapter. The next chapter will tell you all that you would like to know about pronunciation and speaking correctly.

Do invest in a good dictionary so that all your doubts are clarified

Chapter 19

# Report Writing

You have come to know the art of writing letters, CV, and Bed Head Tickets. Each of these requires you to write in a particular manner. Except for informal letters all the others require formal language. One more addition to this list of formal writing is Report Writing. You may get an opportunity at any time in your life to write a report. Here is all that you need to know while writing a report.

At this point you may ask *"How will this help me? Knowing how to write a report?"*"Haven't you, as a student, heard the reading of the college annual report during College Day? Well as you enter your professional life, you will be doing and learning many administerial works. This (report writing) is one of them.

A report can be a two-line hand written memo to a bound volume with any number of pages that may be electronically typed or it may be a volume of computer print–outs. The report may be about an education trip you may have participated, a serious technical meeting, an annual organization report or the report of the annual financial budget of a country. The report may be read out loud publicly or it may be for an individual read. Regardless of the type of report, certain rules/guidelines need to be followed in bringing out a well-done report.

The most important aspect of writing a report is to identify the key facts of a particular matter. After this the matter must be presented in the right order in as simple as possible *format*. So the question arises "what factors are involved in writing a report?"

Writing a report involves a lot of research, trying to get the right words to present the facts, figures to show the gathered statistics the most effective way. All this may sound like a lot of effort to be put in to write a report. All the effort put in will be worth it when the report is printed or read aloud. A well-done report provides detailed information, a good conclusion and recommendations that provide a basis for decisions. The 'terms of reference' of a report direct the writer/writers to cover clearly defined topics like investigating particular product, or an event, company or a proposal. Thus, the terms of reference also decides the kind of report you write.

*Like:*

i. Should it be an investigative report which details the investigation carried out and its findings.

ii. Should it be a recommendatory report which suggests courses of action to be taken in the light of the findings.

iii. Should it be a progressive report which investigates the state of a particular point in a long-term training programme.

Now, this brings us to the question **"What are the parts of a report?"**

In general we can say a report is divided into–

- Title
- Introduction
- Content
- Conclusion
- Recommendation.

If a **report is long and formal** like the annual report of an organization (various departments are **involved**) or the economic budget of a nation, such a report is divided into three main sections. Each section is further divided into relevant components like,

**I Part**

- Title Page
- Objectives/terms of reference
- Table of contents
- List of charts, diagrams & illustrations
- Preface
- Acknowledgements
- Abstract or summary of findings to be detailed in the body of the report.

**II Part** Body of the report/content

- Introduction
- Detailed investigation (if it is needed) and its outcome
- Conclusion+ recommendations

**III Part** Appendices

- Endnotes
- Bibliography
- Supplementary materials like charts and figures.
- Index.

In case your report is not long or you have to write a **short report** that does not exceed four or five pages, then do not follow the scheme suggested above. The principles remain the same but, the report will be divided on general rules containing–

1. Introduction
2. Objective (if any)
3. Content or matter or body of report
4. Conclusion.

Let us now see how we have to go about in writing a report.

The first step is to know who will be the reader or the recipients of your report. If the recipient is the general public the language used and the amount of information provided is different from the recipients who are Board of Directors. The amount of technical information provides changes based on the recipient. No report should be over simplified. This makes the target audience lose interest. Facts and points are omitted based on who the target audience is. One point—you should never put your personal opinions into the report. Your opinions are your own. It is not for public debate. You must present all sides of a question in a balanced and unbiased manner.

The second step is 'research'. You must collect all data available from all the involved sections/ department before starting to write. Here break-up your work into manageable tasks and involve people in helping you to gather the necessary data. Keep in mind the deadline. The amount of time required to collect information should be considered. Make a list of tasks to be done and tick them once they are done.

Third step is storing the information collected. Keep them in an order, either alphabetical (departments) or chronological (which fact/information comes first and so on). When or if you get new ideas jot them down on a notepad. Do not rely on your memory power to come to your aid. Your memory has a lot put into it. Do not confuse it. Put all sheets in a proper file so that you will not lose any single sheet. In case you have to interview (say the senior-most administrative officer) then use a tape recorder so that you won't get their words or the meaning intended wrong or out of context.

Fourth step: This comes only if the report is research-oriented. Use questionnaires to get large scale data. The questionnaire must be specific and detailed and the questions arranged in a logical order. It should not be too long.

Fifth step is drafting the report. You will require several trial drafts before the final report is done. Be patient. Check and recheck to see if you have covered all the vital points. The language used must always be formal. The introduction should be short. The conclusion is done by summarizing your general findings. If a department has solved a problem, a mention is made in the conclusion. Logically, the recommendations section would appear near the end of the report. In special cases where the recommendations have to be incorporated urgently to get results, then they become the main focus of a report and the order of presentation changes.

The title page is very important. Choose the title carefully. Keep it short. But, don't compromise on clarity. Your choice of words should be precise so that the reader will understand immediately.

The terms of reference or objective are always on a new fresh page. It starts with the infinitive form of the verb "to report on" or "to investigate" for example.

The table of contents gives the complete list of the headings and sub-headings along with the page numbers. This gives a complete overview.

A brief preface or foreword is necessary only in case of a long report.

The Acknowledgements Section gives the writer of the report a chance to thank people and institutions that have helped in the research aspect of the report.

While compiling the report, (if it is a long one) you may have referred to a published work (this happens mostly in technical reports) or even quote directly from it. You can mention the original work in a footnote (a note at the foot/end of the page).

Bibliography is given at the end of the report where references to other published works are mentioned with all the details. You can check technical books in your college library. They will all have Bibliography at the end.

Sixth step is putting your sign as the author of the report, whether long or short is immaterial, at the end along with date. If the report has been by a team of people, the team leader or chairman or chairwoman will sign the report and date it.

## Exercises

Here is a sample report writing—an example of a short report writing.

Observe the two pie charts given below. They show the educational profile of employees in the private sector during the years 1955 and 1990. Following is a report made to the employment section of a financial paper on the changing educational scenario and the employment scene and its implication.



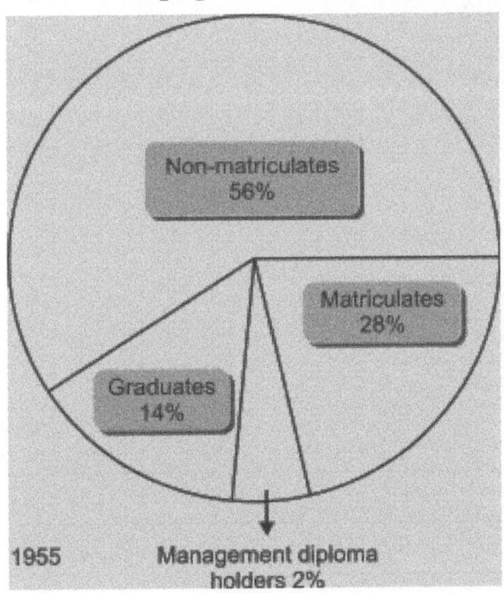


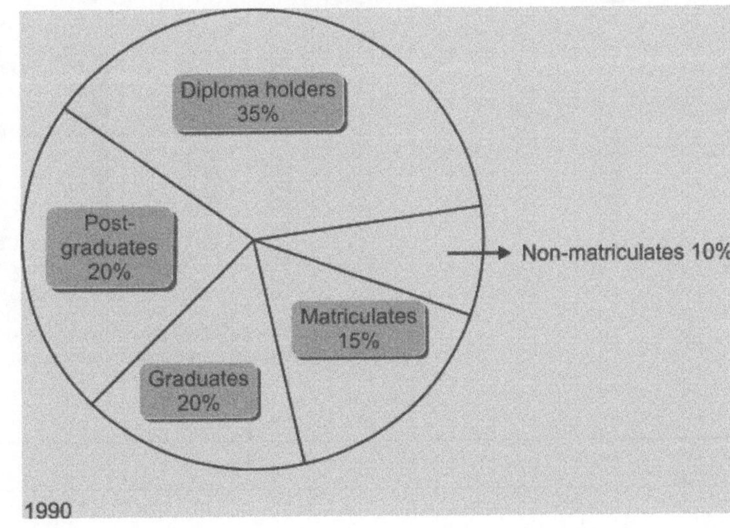


Here is the report:

The huge swing from 2 to 35% in the case of employees with a diploma is quite obvious. Post-graduates being employed in the private sector is a new development. This 20% chunk is significant as it demonstrates that highly qualified employees contribute significantly to the company turnover.These two developments explain the fall in the number of employees with a matriculation (28 to 15%) and non-matriculation ( 56 to 10%) background .

The pie charts clearly show the importance given to education before entering the employment arena which was not the case in the 1950s. It also throws light on why youngsters enter the job arena much later in the 1990s. A significant point to be noted is that the private sector is laying stress on well qualified employees for this change to take place.

## Now try to write similar short length reports for the data given

**I. A vertical bar graph representing two kinds of data is given. The number of students appearing for bank exams and the number of candidates selected over the years is given. The report has to be printed in the national daily newspaper. Prepare a report.**

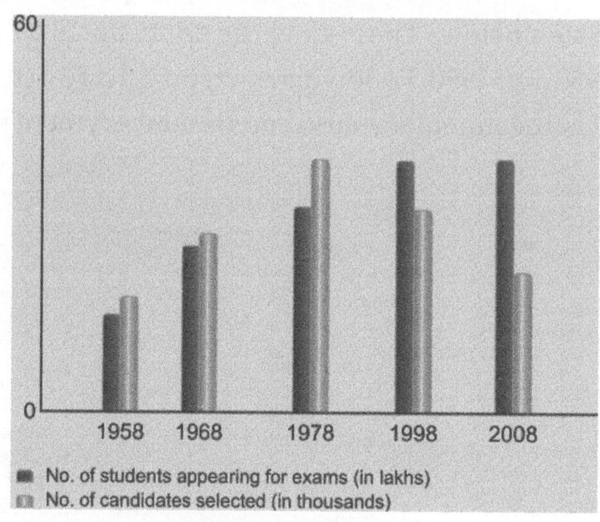

**II. Here is a line graph illustrating the different types of marriage expenditures in India from 1910 to 2010. As a sociologist you have to prepare an analytical report of the marriage trends for a seminar on Indian marriage expenditures.(Expenditure is in rupees ten thousands)**

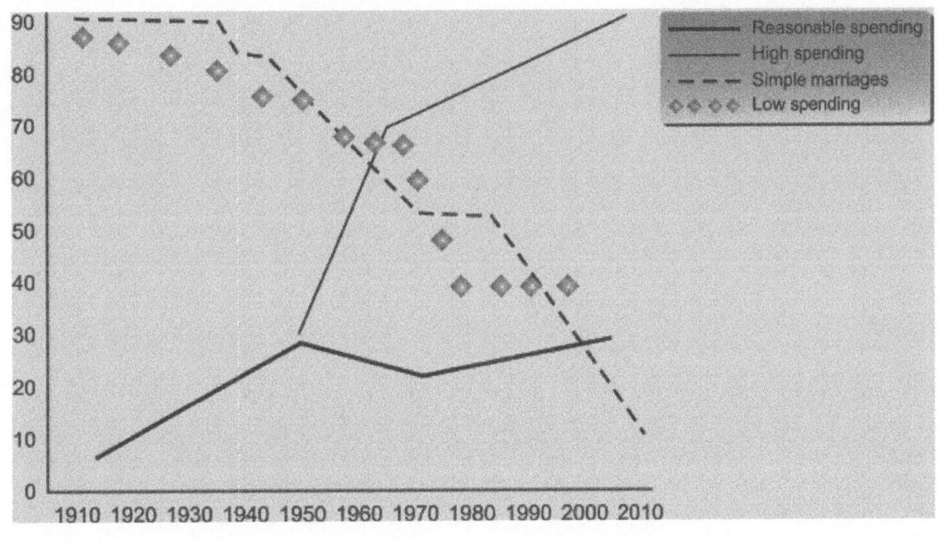


With this we come to the end of report writing. You would have noticed we use indirect speech, past participle form of verbs and past tense form of verbs to do our reports. Practice makes one good in writing reports.

We shall now move onto the next topic.

# Part V

- Am I Speaking Right?
- Spelling Information
- Excercises

# Chapter 20
# Am I Speaking Right?

Millions of foreign students want to learn English as well as they can. But many students want to be able to speak English well, with a pronunciation which can be easily understood. Written English and spoken English are obviously different things. When you can *hear* English properly you can go on and improve your performance.

One of the chief characteristics of human beings is their ability to communicate with their fellow beings. They convey complex messages concerning every aspect of life. A child even at a very early age learns to communicate by imitating the **recurrent sound pattern** she/he has become familiar with. It is only later that she/he learns the visual representation of speech, i.e. writing.

Language starts with the ear. When a baby starts to talk he does it by hearing the sounds his mother makes and imitating them. If a baby is born deaf he cannot hear these sounds and, therefore, cannot imitate them and will not speak. But normal babies can hear and can imitate; they are wonderful imitators, and this gift of imitation lasts for a number of years.

It is well known that a child of ten years or less can learn *any* language perfectly, if it is brought up surrounded by that language, no matter where it was born or who its parents were. But after this age the ability to imitate perfectly becomes less, and adults have great difficulty in mastering the pronunciation (as well as other parts) of foreign languages. Some people are more talented than others; they find pronouncing other languages less difficult, but they never find them easy.

Even though most Indians (some cases Asians and Africans) can use at least two languages as a means of communication, they generally take speech for granted, and seldom stop to think about the complex speech mechanism that makes spoken language possible. So, in this chapter I have tried to give a brief, yes a very brief analysis and description of how sound patterns in English are formed.

If speech depends on hearing fortunately there is a lot of English spoken in the world. In films, on the radio, on tapes, on gramophone records; most people can get the opportunity of listening to English in some way, and this is what you must do. ***You must hear English.*** But just hearing it is not enough; **you must listen to it**, and you must listen to it not for the meaning but for the sound of it. When you are listening to a radio program you will be trying to understand it, but you must try to forget what words mean and listen to the way the words sound.

**Phonetics is the study and science of speech sounds.** When we produce speech sounds we use the speech mechanism which comprises certain organs of the body such as the muscles of the chest, tongue, and the lips and so on. The air that we breathe is modified in different ways to result in various combinations of consonants and vowels. That is probably why speech is popularly known as 'modified breathing'.

The organs of speech and their speech functions can be described with reference to three systems:

**The Respiratory system**

**The Phonatory system,** and

**The Articulatory system.**



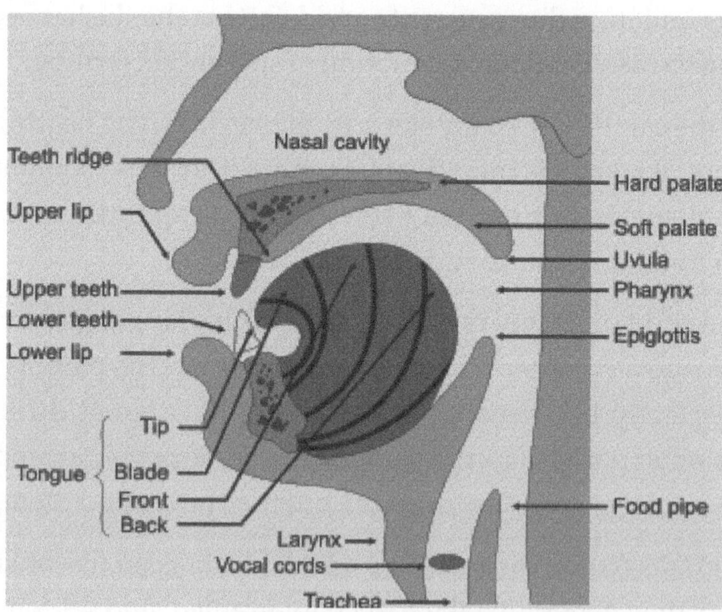


**Fig. 20.1:** Organ of speech

The lungs, the muscles of the chest and the windpipe or trachea are the Organs of Speech belonging to the Respiratory System. The primary function of the lungs as we all know is to enable us to breathe or respire. When the muscles of the chest contract the lungs are compressed and throw the air out.

Besides the lungs there are other organs that can also provide an air stream for the production of speech sounds e.g. **the glottis** and **the velum. The glottalic air stream** is the air stream above the glottis which is closed for the production of sounds using the air stream. Similarly, sounds are produced with the air in front of the **velum** or the soft palate. The passage of air from the lungs is blocked by the back of the tongue which makes firm contact with the velum. This is known as the **Velaric air stream**.

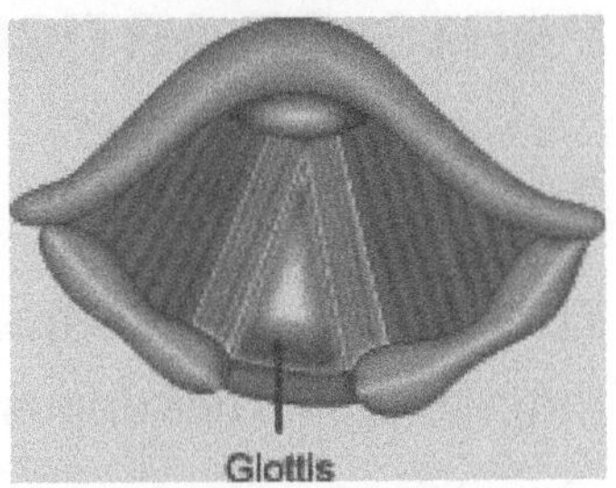


**Fig. 20.2:** Vocal cords drawn wide part

The pulmonic or lung air is used by all the languages of the world. It is the air exhaled from the lungs which initiates the air stream. This air stream mechanism is known as the pulmonic aggressive air stream mechanism when the air which is breathed initiates the air stream for speech production.

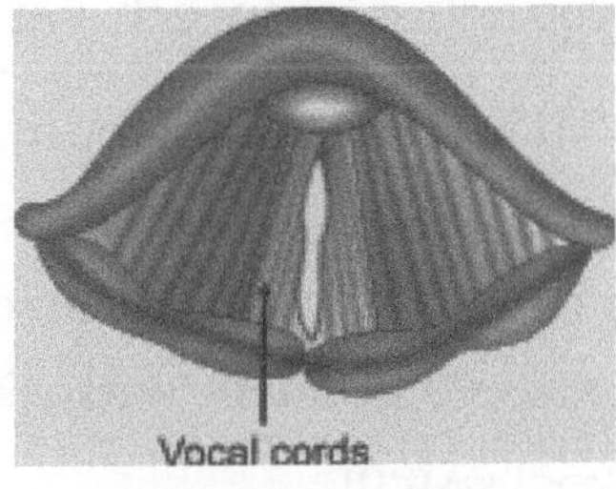


**Fig. 20.3:** Vocal cords held loosely together

The phonatory system is comprised of the larynx in the throat. You know as nursing students that the larynx is a muscular structure. The front part of this structure can be felt in the neck, and is commonly known as the 'Adam's Apple'. The Adam's apple is more prominent in men than in women.

The larynx contains a pair of muscular bands or folds called **the Vocal cords**. These are placed horizontally from front to back, joined at the front but separated at the back. The space between the cords is called **the Glottis**.

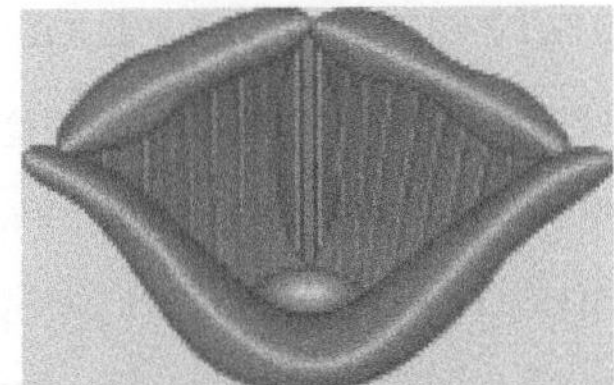

**Fig. 20.4:** Vocal cords held tightly together

Three positions:

1. Held wide apart
2. Held loosely together
3. Held tightly together.

After passing through the larynx the air is further modified by the various shapes that the articulatory above the larynx assume, before it meets the air outside. Each modification affects the quality of the sound produced. These articulators together constitute **the Articulatory System**.

## PARTS OF ARTICULATORY SYSTEM

### a. The Pharynx

The Pharynx extends from the top of the larynx to the root of the tongue (the hinder-most part of the tongue) which lies opposite it.

### b. The Lips

The lips, which are in the front-most position of the oral tract, have an important part to play in the production of speech sounds.

It is obvious that the lips can take up various different positions. They can be brought firmly together as in /p/ or /b/ or /m/ so that they completely block the mouth; the lower lip can be drawn inward and slightly upwards to touch the upper front teeth as in the sounds/f/ and /v/. And they can be kept apart either flat or with different amounts of rounding, and they can be pushed forward to a greater or lesser extent.

Of course, the closed position for /p, b, m/ and the lip-teeth position for /f/ and /v/ are used in English, but apart from this the English do not move their lips with very much energy as is done in most Asian languages: their lips are never very far apart, they do not take up very rounded shapes, they are rarely spread very much and almost never pushed forward or protruded. Watch English people and American people talk either in real life or on films and notice how little the lips and the lower jaw move; some people make more lip movement than others, but it is never necessary to exaggerate these movements. Watch people talking your language too, and see whether they move their lips more than the English or the Americans. If so, you must remember when talking English to use lips less than you do in your own language. The same is true for movements of the jaw: in normal speech there is rarely more than half an inch between the lips or a quarter of an inch between the teeth even when the mouth is at its widest open.

### c. The Teeth

We produce some consonants with the help of the teeth. The initial consonant sounds in the English words *think, that* are produced by placing the tip of the tongue between the upper teeth and the lower teeth and the initial consonants in the English words *fan, van* are produced by placing the upper teeth very tightly on the lower lip.

The lower front teeth are not important in speech except that if they are missing certain sounds, e.g. /s/ and /z/ will be difficult to make. But the two upper front teeth are used in English to some extent.

## d. The Teeth Ridge

The teeth ridge or the **alveolar ridge** is the convex part of the roof of the mouth lying just behind the upper teeth. This hard, raised structure can be felt with the tip of the tongue. Many consonant sounds are produced at the teeth ridge.

## The Hard Palate

Beyond the alveolar ridge is a hard bony surface which we can feel if we move our tongue from the alveolar ridge along the roof of the mouth. Some sounds are produced at the hard palate. The initial sound in the English word *Yes* is produced this way.

## The Soft Palate

If we continue to move our tongue it cannot go beyond the point in the roof of the mouth where bony structure ends and the roof of the mouth becomes soft. This soft portion of the roof of the mouth is known as the **soft palate** or **the velum**.

## The Palate

The palate, as figure shows, forms the roof of the mouth and separates the mouth cavity from the nose (or nasal) cavity. Make the tip of your tongue touch as much of your own palate as you can: most of it is hard and fixed in position, but when your tongue-tip is as far back as it will go, away from your teeth, you will notice that the palate becomes soft.

You can easily see the soft part of the palate if you use a mirror: turn your back to the light, open your mouth wide and say the vowel /a:/, and move the mirror so that the light shines into your mouth. You will be able to see the soft palate curving down towards the tongue and becoming narrower as it does so until it ends in a point called *the uvula* /ju:vjula/. Behind the soft palate you will be able to see part of the back wall of the pharynx. The soft palate can move: it can be raised so that it makes a firm contact with the back wall of the pharynx and this stops the breath from going up into the nasal cavity

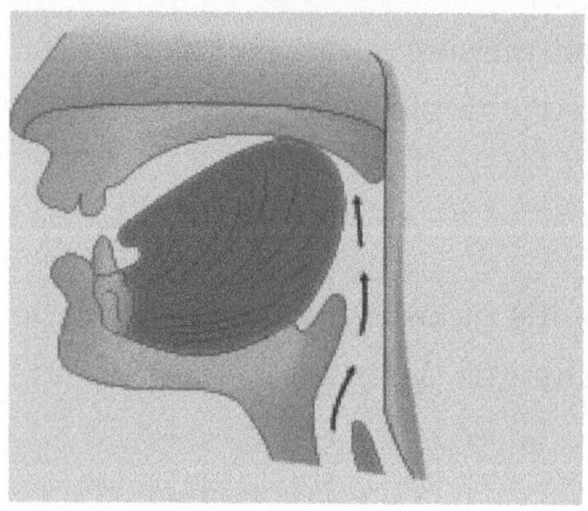

Fig. 20.5: Velar closure and velic closure

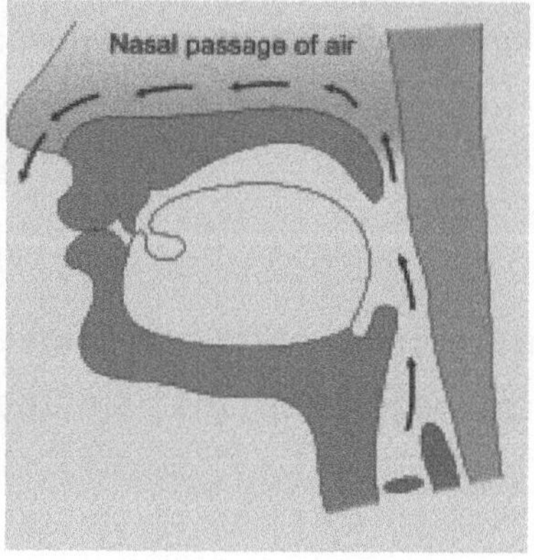


Fig. 20.6: Nasal passage open; oral passage closed

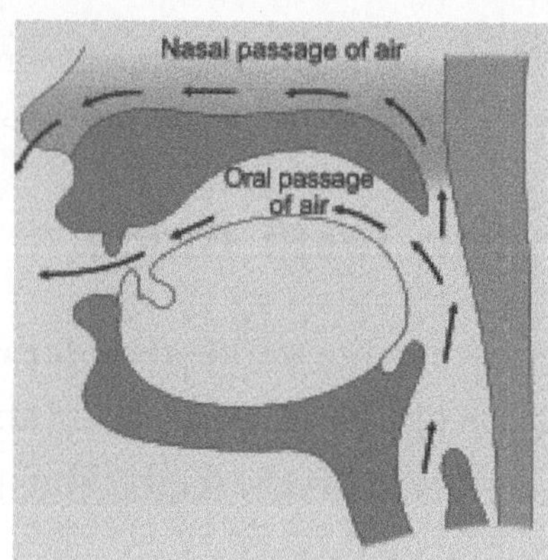


Fig. 20.7: Nasal passage open; oral passage also open



and forces it to go into the mouth only. You can see this raising of the soft palate in your mirror if you keep your mouth wide open in position for the vowel /a:/ and push out your breath very fast, as if you were trying to blow out a match, still with your mouth open wide. You will see the soft palate move quickly upwards so that the breath all comes out of the mouth and none of it goes up into the nasal cavity. And when you relax after this the soft palate will come down again into its lowered position.

As such, therefore, a speech sound can be studied at three stages- **the production stage**, **the transmission stage** and **the reception stage**.

## The Tongue

The tongue is the most important of the organs of speech because it has the greatest variety of movement. Although the tongue has no obvious natural divisions like the palate, it is useful to think of it as divided into four parts.

The *back* of the tongue lies under the soft palate when the tongue is at rest; the *front* lies under the hard palate, the *tip* and the *blade* lie under the alveolar ridge, the tip being the most forward part of all and the blade between the tip and the front. The tip and blade are particularly mobile and, as we have seen, they can touch the whole of the lips, the teeth, the alveolar ridge and the hard palate. The front can be flat on the bottom of the mouth or it can be raised to touch the hard palate, or it can be raised to any extent between these two extremes. Say the vowel /a:/ again and front rises a little; now say /e/ as in *met* (still keep your mouth as wide open as you can): the front rises again; and if you go on to say

/i:/ as in *see* you will see that the front rises to a very high position, so high that it is hidden behind the teeth. For /i:/ the front of the tongue comes vey close to the hard palate. Put your mouth in this position, for /i:/, and draw air *inwards* quickly; you will feel cold air on the front of the tongue and on the hard palate just above it.

Before we proceed with the description and classification of speech sounds, we need to understand the categories- 'vowel' and ' consonant' and define them satisfactorily.

Vowel and consonants are popularly defined with reference to the letters of the alphabet. Remember the letters a, e, i, o, u are called 'vowels' and the rest are 'consonants'. This definition is misleading because **'vowel' and 'consonant' are essentially categories of speech sounds**. When we label the letters of the alphabet as 'vowel' and 'consonant' we probably do it on the basis of the assumption that there is perfect correspondence between the letters and the sounds they stand for. This correspondence, unfortunately, is not perfect in any language, least of all in English.

'Vowel' and 'Consonant' are also defined in **phonetic** and **linguistic** terms. When we define them in phonetic terms, we do so with reference to their production, when we define them in linguistic terms, we refer to their function in a given language.

In phonetic terms, a vowel is a sound for whose production the oral passage is unobstructed, so that the air can flow from the lungs to the lips and beyond without being stopped, without having to squeeze through a narrow construction, which would cause audible friction.

A consonant, on the other hand, is a sound for whose production the air current is completely stopped, or is forced through a narrow constriction which causes audible friction.

**Then you may ask "so the definitions you learnt earlier is it wrong?" No. It is not. The new definition you are reading now about vowels and consonants are purely as Phonetic terms. The earlier definition at the beginning of the book is correct for students learning the English language.**

Let us look at a few examples. For example the English word *bar*. The vowel represented by letters *ar*, is produced with the mouth wide open and the tongue low in mouth. The air passage is unobstructed and the air passes into the atmosphere outside without any friction. The sound is, therefore, called a vowel. The sound represented by the letter *b* is produced by a complete closure of the oral passage of air at the two lips, and then the sudden release of air held behind the closure. Thus, there is an obstruction, for a while, to the flow of air from the lungs. Because of this obstruction the resultant sound is regarded as a consonant.

*Example*: The English word *see*. The sound represented by the letter *ee* is produced by raising the front of the tongue fairly high, so that the passage between the tongue and the hard palate is fairly narrow but not narrow enough to cause any audible friction in the sound produced. The sound is therefore, regarded as a vowel. In the production of the s-sound in the English word *see*, the tip and blade of the tongue rise so high towards the teeth ridge that the passage of air is very narrow and the air passes out with audible friction. Thus the sound is a consonant.

Let us take the initial sounds in the English words *yell* and *wind*. In the production of these sounds there is no obstruction to the air flow and no narrowing to cause audible friction. The two sounds, in phonetic terms must therefore be regarded as vowels. But the English language regards them as consonants, because they function as consonants. They always occupy the position of consonants in English words, and take the article *a*, rather then *an* before them unlike English vowels. Thus we get *a yell*, *a wind* not *an yell* or *an wind*.



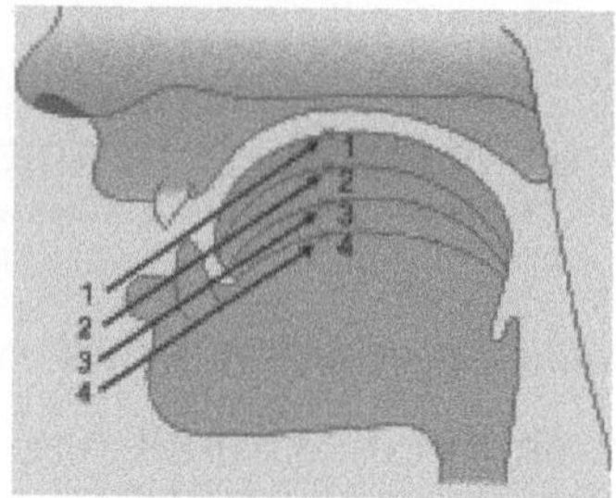


**Fig. 20.8:** Tongue positions for the four front vowels

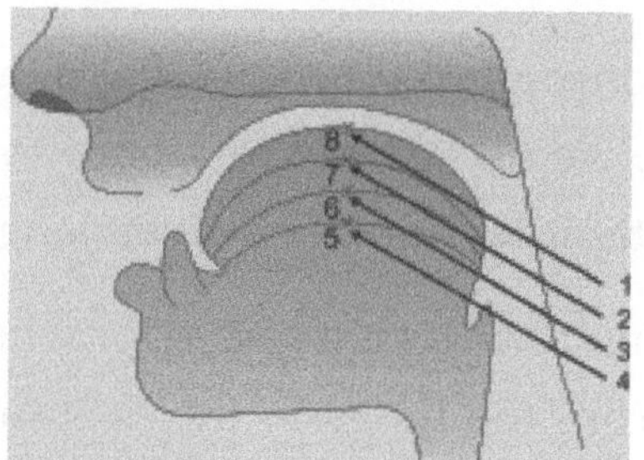


**Fig. 20.9:** Tongue positions for the four back vowels

## Sounds and Sound-Groups

A sound is made by definite movements of the organs of speech, and if those movements are exactly repeated the result will always be the same sound; it is easy to show that there are more than forty-four sounds in English – even in the pronunciation of a single person, without worrying about differences between people.

When we pronounce the words *he, hat, who, hi:*, haet, hu:, the /h/-sounds are different: in pronouncing /h/ we put our mouth into the position needed for the following vowel and then push out air through this position, but since the three different vowels have three different mouth-positions it follows that the three /h/-sounds must also be different.

In all languages we speak with air from the lungs. We draw it into the lungs quickly and we release it slowly and then interfere with its passage in various ways and at various places.

## The Vocal Cords

The air released by the lungs comes up through the wind-pipe and arrives first at *the larynx.* The larynx contains two small bands of elastic tissue, which can be thought of as two flat strips of rubber, lying opposite each other across the air passage. These are the vocal cords.

The inner edges of the vocal cords can be moved towards each other so that they meet and completely cover the top of the wind-pipe, or they can be drawn apart so that there is a gap between them (known as *the glottis*) through which the air can pass freely: this is their usual position when we breathe quietly in and out.

When the vocal cords are brought together tightly no air can pass through them and if the lungs are pushing air from below this air is compressed. If the vocal cords are then opened suddenly the compressed air bursts out with a sort of coughing noise.

If the vocal cords are brought together quite gently, the air from the lungs will be able to force them apart for a moment, but then they will return to the closed position; then the air will force them apart again, and they will close again, and so on. This is a very rapid process and may take place as many as 800 times per second. It is obviously not possible to hear a musical note. The height of the note depends on the speed of opening and closing of the vocal cords; if they open and close very quickly the note will be high, if they open and close slowly the note will be low. The note, whether high or low, produced by this rapid opening and closing of the vocal cords is called *voice.*

The sounds which are not voiced – *voiceless* sounds – are made with the vocal cords drawn apart so that the air can pass out freely between them and there is no vibration. The difference between voiced and voiceless can be used to distinguish between what are otherwise similar sounds. Say a long /s/-sound again, and in the middle of it turn the voice on: this will give you a /z/-sound, buzzing rather than hissing. But not all the voiced sounds of English have similar voiceless sounds, for example the voiceless /m/-sound which you made just now does not occur in English, and even when there are pairs of similar sounds which are voiced and voiceless this may not be the only difference between them, as we shall see later.

Immediately above the larynx is a space behind the tongue and reaching up towards the nasal cavity: this space is called *the pharynx* /faerinks/.

Now as nursing students you already know how complex the functioning of the human body is and the treatment of it when things go wrong. The above explanation of how speech sounds are produced will make you feel how lucky one is to have a normal functioning of vocal chords. The magnitude of all that the deaf and dumb miss, is felt here.

## Facts

If you can hear a hum during the production of the sound, the vocal cords are vibrating and the sound is **voiced.** If no hum or buzz can be heard then the vocal cords are not vibrating and the sound being produced is **voiceless.**

If the soft palate is raised to shut off the nasal passage, there is a velic closure, during which only oral sounds can be produced. If the soft palate is lowered, there is no velic closure, and therefore either nasal or nasalized sounds can be produced.

**The point or place of articulation** is determined by the passive articulator. For example, if the front of the tongue (active articulator) is raised towards the hard palate (passive articulator) to make a complete closure or for a narrowing of the air passage, then the place of articulation is the palate, and the sound is **palatal** sound.

**The manner of articulation** refers to the kind of closure or narrowing involved in the production of the initial sound in the English word butter, the two lips make a complete closure.

Let us consider the main places of articulation of consonants beginning with the front most articulators.

**a.** ***Bilabial***: Those consonants in the articulation of which the upper and lower lips are involved. For example, the initial sounds in the English words, *post, boast, meal, win.*

**b.** **Labio-dental**: Those consonants in the production of which the active articulator is the lower lip and the passive articulator is the upper teeth. The initial consonants in the English words *fate* and *vow* are labio-dental consonants.

**c.** **Dental** consonants are those in the production of which the active articulator is the tip of the tongue and the passive articulator the upper teeth. Examples of dental consonants are the initial consonants in the English words, *thin* and *these.*

**d.** **Alveolar** consonants are produced with the blade of the tongue as the active articulator and the teeth ridge as the passive articulator. For example, the initial consonants in the English words *tool, day, lip, nail, sit, zoo.*

e. **Post alveolar** consonants are those in the production of which the active articulator is the tip of the tongue, and the passive articulator the rear part of the teeth ridge. For example, the initial consonant of the English word *red*.

f. **Retroflex** consonants are produced with the underside of the tip of the tongue as the articulator and front of the hard palate as the passive articulator.

g. **Palato- alveolar**: For the production of palate-alveolar consonants (i) the blade of the tongue as the active articulator, articulates against the teeth ridge which is the passive articulator. At the same time the front of the tongue (active articulator) is raised towards the hard palate (passive articulator). For example the initial consonants in the English words *chop, just, ship*, and the sound represented by the spelling *si* in the words *provision, revision*.

h. **Palatal** consonants are produced with the front of the tongue as the active articulator and the hard palate as passive articulator. For example, the initial consonant in the English word *yard*.

i. **Velar**: For the production of velar consonants the active articulator, the back of the tongue articulates against the passive articulator, the soft palate. For example, the final consonants in the English words *rock, bag, ting*

j. **Uvular**: The active articulator in the production of uvular consonants is the back of the tongue, and the passive articulator the uvula.

k. **Pharyngeal**: The active articulator for the production of these consonants is the hindermost part of the tongue and the wall of the pharynx. An example of a pharyngeal consonant is the Arabic consonant represented by the spelling *h* in the word *Mohammed*. This consonant does not occur in English and most of the Indian languages.

l. **Glottal:** The articulators for the glottal sounds are the two cords which move closer resulting in a narrowing of the air passage. For example, the initial consonants in the English word *hat*.

   i. **Plosive**: In the production of a plosive there is a complete closure of the articulators at some point in the vocal tract thus completing shutting off the air passage. For example, the initial sounds in the English words *pit, bit, tip, dip, keep, goal* are plosives- two are bilabial plosives, two alveolar plosives and two velar plosives, respectively.

   ii. **Affricate**: Affricates are produced by a complete closure of the air passage, followed by the building up of pressure behind the closure, and the gradual release of the blocked air. For example, the initial sounds in the English words *choice* and *joy*.

iii. **Nasal**: Nasals are those consonants in the production of which there is a complete closure of the oral passage while the nasal passage remains open, so that the air passes freely through the nose. For example, the medial sounds in the English words *simmer, sinner, singer* (represented by the spelling *mm, nn, ng*) are nasal consonants.

iv. **Trill or Roll** consonants produced by the intermittent taps of the active articulator against the passive articulator are called Trills or Rolls. No closure is involved in the production of these sounds. English does not have any Trills or Rolls. However, in an extended and emphatic articulation of the intial sound in the English words red, round for example, the resultant sound will be a Trill or a Roll.

v. **Flap**: Where the production of a roll consists of several taps of the active articulator against the passive articulator, the production of a flap involves only a single tap of the active articulator against the passive articulator.

vi. **Lateral**: In the production of a lateral, though the center of the oral tract is closed owning to a contact between the active and the passive articulator at some point in the vocal tract, the air escapes from the sides of the contact.

vii. **Fricative**: To produce a fricative there is no closure made anywhere, there is only a narrowing. The active articulator moves towards the passive articulator at some point in the vocal tract, so that there is a very narrow gap for the air to pass through. This causes audible friction. For example, the initial sounds in the English words below are fricatives: *face, veil, think, those, see, zebra, sheep, have.*

viii. **Frictionless continuant**: Unlike fricatives (for the production of which the degree of narrowing is enough to cause audible friction in the sound produced) frictionless continuants are produced by a lesser degree of narrowing of the articulators so that the air passes out freely and no audible friction accompanies the sound produced.

ix. **Semi- vowel**: semi-vowels are vowel –like in phonetic form but function as consonants. For example, the initial consonants in the English words *weight* and *yawn*.

In the production of a vowel, there is no obstruction to the air in the pharynx and the mouth, nor is there any narrowing to the extent that it causes audible friction. Vowels generally have a 'hum' when produced. In other words, vowels are normally **voiced.**

The parts of the tongue that are involved in the production of vowels are the **front** of the tongue which lies opposite the hard palate, the **back** of the tongue which lies opposite the **soft palate** when it is at rest, and the **center** of the tongue which lies opposite the back of the hard palate and the front of the soft palate. The center of the tongue is hard to determine and is imagined. The vowels produced when each of these parts of the tongue is raised are called **front, back and central** respectively. For example, the vowels in the English words *neat, knit, net* are front vowels. The vowels in the English words *card, cod, cord, could, cooed* are back vowels. And the vowels in the English words *bud, bird* are central vowels.

In the production of vowels any part of the tongue can be raised, but the height to which it can be raised is restricted so that there is no audible friction. Also any part of the tongue can be lowered, but not beyond a certain point for the production of vowels. The vowels produced when any part of the tongue is raised to the highest point are called **close** vowels. Those vowels produced with any part of the tongue at the lowest point are called **open** vowels.

The lips can thus be spread as for the vowels in the English word *feel*: **neutral** as for the vowel in the English word *fur:* **open** for the vowel in *far:* **open-rounded** for the vowel in *rod* and **close-rounded** for the vowel in *rude.* It is the general practice to regard the spread, neutral and open positions as **unrounded** and the other two positions as **rounded.**

The tongue remains unchanged throughout the process of their production. These sounds, in other words are called **monophthongs** or pure vowels.

The movement of the tongue from one position to another is so gradual and smooth that it may be called a glide. The vowels produced as a result of such glides are called **diphthongs**. Diphthongs are not the same as a sequence of two monophthongs example, the vowels in the English word *seeing* are a sequence of two monophthongs, whereas the vowel in the English word *fear* is a diphthong.

As mentioned in the beginning of this chapter, listening to English through different means helps, there are some disadvantages.

You can stop recorded films, radio programs, gramophone records and tapes and hear them. With them you can repeat any part of the text as often as you need, and you must do this: it is much better for your ear if you listen to the same passage six times than if you listen to six different passages; but be careful – listen closely each time, don't relax after two or three hearings, try to keep your ears as closely concentrated on the sound of the passage at the sixth hearing as at the first. In this way you will build up a store of sound-memory which will form a firm base for your performance.

When you practice (aloud) you must listen carefully and accurately. If you have listened properly in the first place you will know what the English words and sentences sound like, and you must compare as closely as you can the sounds that come out of your mouth with the sounds that you are holding in your head, in your sound-memory. Don't be satisfied too easily, try to match your sounds exactly with the sounds that you have listened to.

If you can, record on the tape-recorder a sentence or a longer passage with which you are familiar through hearing it said by an English speaker. Then listen to it, closely and carefully, and see where your performance does not match the original; mark the places where you are dissatisfied, and practice these bits until you think you have them right; then record the passage, listen critically again, and repeat the sequence. One word of warning – a tape-recorder will not do the job for you; it is a useful instrument, but it is not a magic wand which will make your English perfect without any effort from you.

If you are interested to know more, a book on Phonetics will guide you. This is just a brief introduction. With this, we enter the next interesting chapter—All About Spellings.

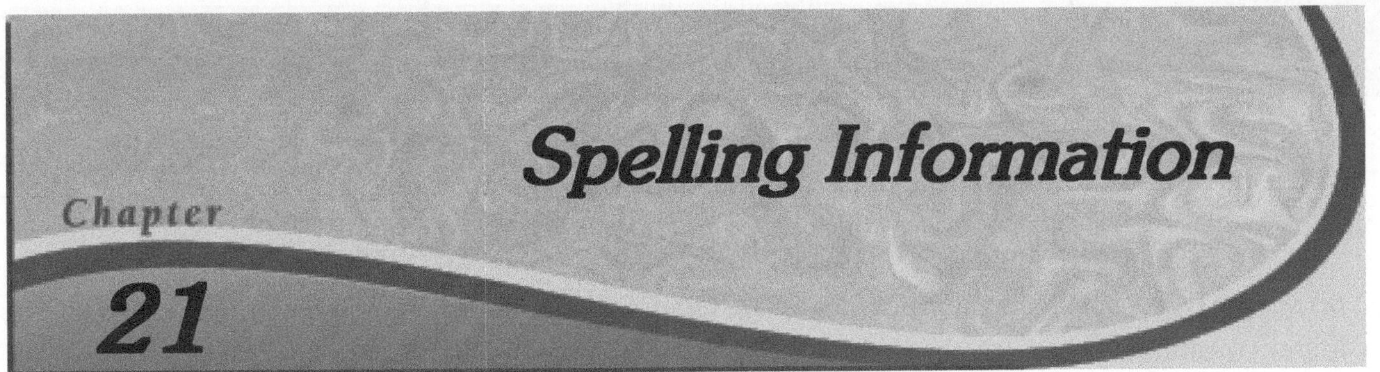


In the previous chapter you understood the production of sound of the English words. The few techniques of practise that help you in becoming familiar with English language have also been given.

Speaking or talking and writing are different forms of communication. One of the ways of going wrong in written communication is not knowing the correct spelling of the words you are using.

This brings us to the question "What is spelling?"

Spell means to write letters of a word (Names - Proper nouns are included) in their correct order or the accepted order.

Spelling is the ability of a person to spell. It can also be described as the action or process of forming words correctly from letters.

*Example*

C-A-T is cat

R-E-T-I-C-E-N-T is reticent

The letters in Roman capitals demonstrate the correct order of letters of the words given beside it. You may ask "Is this exclusive to the English language?"

No it is not. Every language that has a script (that is letters) has a defined spelling pattern. Here we will limit ourselves to English language only.

Confusion is created when spellings are not done the right way or when the word is used in a sentence that does not suit it. You may wonder at this statement. Let me show you how confusions occur.

*Example*: Let us take the word 'Spell'.

Look at the two sentences given below.

i. The magician recited a spell.

ii. How do you spell your name?

Which one is right? You will say (ii) based on the explanation given above.

Well, any person who knows English language well, will say, both are right.

You see the word 'spell' has different meanings. Open a dictionary and you will come to know all the different meanings.

Thus, here in (i) Spell means "words which when spoken are thought to have magical power.

*See these two words.*

Know/No

Both the words are pronounced the same. So, which do you use when? If you don't give attention to a minute detail like this, confusions occur.

To remove these confusions let us first introduce ourselves to the wonderful world of words.

***Words which have unique characteristics are classified as—***

1. Homophones
2. Homonyms
3. Synonyms
4. Antonyms
5. Compound words
6. Prefixes
7. Suffixes

Let us get to know all these interesting words.

**Homophones** are those words which have the same pronunciation but different spellings and meanings.

***Example***

Some Sum

Knew New

Here 'Some' gives the meaning of a few and 'Sum' is arithmetical calculation.

*Knew* is the past tense of know and new is any product or material that is introduced, seen, invented for the first time. It also means unused.

**Homonyms** are those words which have the same pronunciation and spelling, but the meaning changes.

***Example***

Light

**One meaning** of light is a kind of natural radiation that makes things visible.

*The light of the sun.*

**Second meaning** is flame or spark. Have you got a light? (for cigarette)

**Third meaning** is understanding or enlightenment.

**Synonyms** are words which have similar meanings in the same language.

*Example:* Slay, kill, murder are synonyms.

**Antonyms** are the words which are opposite in meaning to another word.

*Example*: Old - Young, new

**Compound** words have been dealt with in the chapter Nouns.

**Prefix:** When one or more letters are added at the beginning of a word to add or change the meaning of that word, such letters are called as prefixes.

Co- ,ex-, non-, pre-, re- are some prefixes.

*Example*: un in unhappy

re in remade

**Suffix:** When one or more letters are added at the end of a word to make another word, such letters are called as Suffixes.

*Example:* *y* in rusty

*en* in strengthen.

*Note:* Prefix and Suffix are not hyphenated words like compound words.

## Exercises

**I. Form compound words from the given words:**

| | | | | | | | |
|---|---|---|---|---|---|---|---|
| moon | never | under | light | of | chess | power | escape |
| the | take | man | board | arm | post | war | bird |
| chair | man | rail | fire | jail | way | horse | less |

_______________ _______________ _______________ _______________

_______________ _______________ _______________ _______________

_______________ _______________ _______________ _______________

**II. Write the homophones of the following:**

night _______________

rite _______________

son _______________

sweet _______________

soot _______________

knot _______________

board _______________

so _______________

shake _______________

grate _______________

dye _______________

**III. Write the different uses of the following homonyms:**

| | |
|---|---|
| Bill | Fork |
| Pitcher | Jar |
| Pictures | Just |
| Dump | Knob |
| Eve | Miss |
| Faint | Order |

**4. Give the synonyms of:**

Circular

Attorney

Belie

______________________________

Dirty

______________________________

Enate

______________________________

Fad

______________________________

Grassland

______________________________

Hideous

______________________________



Interloper

______________________________

Jay

______________________________

**V. Give the antonyms of:**

Day ____________ Keep ____________ Top ____________

Calm ____________ Black ____________ Inside ____________

War ____________ Fair ____________ Sit ____________

Love ____________ Up ____________ Happy ____________

Married ____________ Front ____________ Laugh ____________

Understand ____________

**VI. Make a list of prefixes and suffixes from the data given below:**

-a mis in

be ab er ar ed er

to or

un under dom

yer ful y

ly ward ish

ness

hood en less ful

| | | | | | | | |
|---|---|---|---|---|---|---|---|
| bed | time | night | tie | charge | paint | gold | silver |
| child | gift | copper | help | board | deed | kind | do |
| go | beg | girl | learn | jar | lead | holy | fold |
| ground | sail | room | woman | need | side | day | true |
| sell | use | free | bold | chat | joy | man | for |
| back | out | dirt | wind | | | | |

______________________________________________

______________________________________________

______________________________________________

______________________________________________

______________________________________________

______________________________________________

This chapter may make you take up your dictionary and use it again and again. This will help you to build up your vocabulary. As you will flip through the dictionary you come across words that have a German or Latin or French or Greek written beside them. This is intriguing and you may begin to wonder at the connection of all these European languages on English.

Here is a small introduction to the formation of words in English. You may feel like asking why would you need to know this. The answer is simple. Being a student nurse you are exposed to various words. Some the moment you read it feels anything but English. Like scientific terms, Latin names. At such times, if you know why or how it has been accepted in the English language, understanding becomes easier and then learning it and using it in a sentence becomes easier.

Words that are not derived or compounded or developed from other words are called as **Primary Words.**

From these Primary Words other kinds of words are formed. They are:

1. Compound Words
2. Primary Derivatives
3. Secondary Derivatives



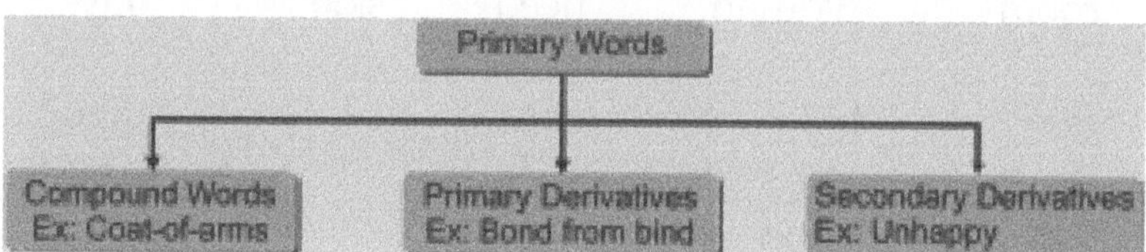


1. **Compound Words** are formed by joining two or more simple words.

   *Example:* Moonlight, man-of-war

2. **Primary Derivatives** are formed by making some change in the body of the simple word.

   *Example:* Bond from bind, breach from break

3. **Secondary Derivatives** are formed by an addition to the beginning or the end of the word-

   Prefixes and Suffixes.

   *Example:* Unhappy, goodness.

*Under this, there are:*

i. English Prefixes

ii. Latin Prefixes

iii. Greek Prefixes

iv. English Suffixes

v. Latin Suffixes

vi. Greek Suffixes

Examples are:

i. aboard, ashore, beside, income, misjudge, overflow, to-night, unholy.

ii. abuse, adjoin, ambiguous, anticipate, ancestor, benefit, biscuit.

iii. analysis, apology, architect, catalogue, dilemma, dysentery, emblem.

iv. painter, martyrdom, womanhood, wedlock, boldness, hatred, lordship.

v. artisan, scholar, advocate, marriage, punishment, frailty.

vi. cynic, chemist, obelisk, enthusiasm, crisis.

There are many more words. As you go through a good Standard English dictionary you will come across more.

Some words are retained from the original language in English. Such words are called as **Root Words.**

| Example: Corpus | We get Corpse, Corporation, This is from Latin language. | Corpulent from this root word. |
|---|---|---|
| Geo | We get Geology, Geography, This is from Greek language. | Geometry from this root word. |

With this we come to the end of this book. But, learning never stops. The more you practise the better you do. The more you read, listen and speak, the more knowledge you acquire (you acquire better understanding of the language). Getting to know the language throws interesting information about the language you are studying. As influences seep in from other languages to English it grows. This is true of all languages in this world.

Welcome to the world of knowledge as I bid good-bye to you.

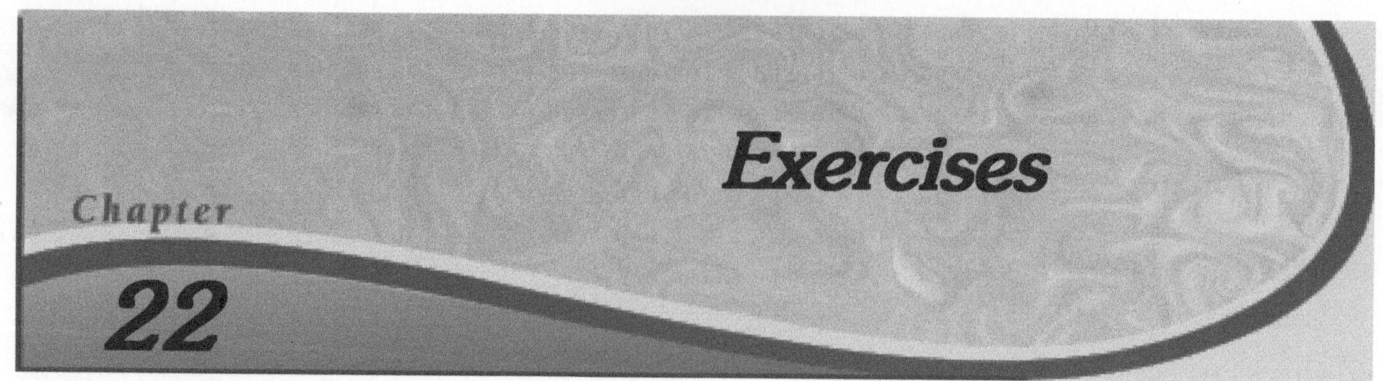

# Chapter 22 Exercises

After going through the entire book you are now in a position to understand the mistakes you and others make in speech and writing. You are now filled with a burgeoning excitement to put into effect your new found knowledge and prowess in using English language. So here are a few extra exercises to help you realize that dream. You may be able to assess yourself and laugh at your mistakes. So enjoy doing these exercises all by yourself.

## 1. Fill in the blanks with the suitable prepositions

i. France is famous ____________ its perfumes.

ii. The pig subsists __________ the coarsest _______ food.

iii. Archie is fond _____ architecture.

iv. It is natural in every human being _____ wish _____ recognition.

v. The speaker is evidently enamoured ___ the subject.

vi. Ambition does not always help ____ achieve ultimate happiness.

vii. Newly acquired freedom is sometimes liable _____ abuse.

viii. The little boy proved quite a handful ____ the nurse.

ix. The software engineer knows his subject well, but is totally ignorant _____ manners.

x. The income derived ______ the ownership ____ a house is commonly called rent.

xi. That old man is afflicted __________ leprosy.

xii. They have an unquenched appetite ____ pursuing knowledge.

xiii. Their enmity ________ the seniors cost them heavily _______ the college.

xiv. I am in charge _____ the general ward .

xv. Access ____ the library is denied to the repeated offenders.

xvi. She is accustomed ____ luxury.

xvii. Dr Ray was somewhat susceptible ____ flattery.

xviii. ________________ time the student realized his mistake.

xix. It is tough ____ work ____________ the parameters.

xx. The garden is designed __________ the building.

xxi. Rahul participated in the race _________ Roy.

xxii. ___________ his attitude , he estranged his friends.

xxiii. ____________ the principal I read the college report.

xxiv. ____________ rope they climbed the rocky face of the mountain.

xxv. The child talked _____________ the parent's instructions.

xxvi. ________________ his researches he met many people.

xxvii. ____________ talking, prove your worth by doing something worthwhile.

xxviii. The little girl performed her dance well ____________ an audience.

xxx. The court gave the ruling _________________ the doctor.

## 2. Write the following paragraphs in indirect speech

"What do you want?"he said to her.

"Some money to buy food" she said.

"Why don't you work and earn some money?" he shouted.

"No one will give me one "she said.

_______________________________________________

_______________________________________________

_______________________________________________

_______________________________________________

"Do you really come from China?" said the prince.

"Yes. Your highness. I do." said the man.

"How do people look, dress and eat in China?" asked the prince.

"As all people do your highness" said the man.

"Have you anything else to tell me?" asked the doctor.

"I feel like vomiting just before eating food" said the girl.

"Since when have you felt this way?" said the doctor.

"Three days" said the girl.

"Good evening mam" said Siri.

"Good evening Siri "said mam. "Haven't the others come yet?"

"No mam. I am always the first to come. It is boring to wait for others" said Siri.

"Yes. It is Siri. I hope the others will not make a habit to come late. Let me talk to them" said mam.

# Excercises

Doctor in the ward to a nurse:

Doctor: Sister, have the results come?

Sister: Yes Sir.

Doctor: Put up a diabetic chart. I have prescribed insulin. Make a note. He has to be given twice a day after blood sugar check-up.

**3. Correct the mistakes in the following sentences and rewrite them in the space provided**

The hill going up, an house old seen.

I meeting friend in park.

The medical representative come into clinic.

All nursing came students to party.

Travelling to Delhi Rajadhani by beautiful experience is express.

Night is the cold winter in.

Morning morning why you shouting like this ya?

She not noing English talking.

In a follow-up visit this conversation took place.

Doctor: How are you?

Patient: Oh! Doctor I'm better. My fever has subsidized. But still my nose is soaring.

I laughing laughing not speaking. Only laugh laugh. All seeing me laugh also.

I putted the glass things in basket.Right know?

Eating eating they all talking talking my head aching.

This portion of the exercises leads you to writing conversations. When you are able to do this, you can be sure that you are able to visualize English and thereby speak the same well.

**4. Fill the blank spaces in the following conversations (Yes you have to use your imagination. Only request that do not let your imagination run away with you)**

Imagine you have received a telephone call and complete the conversation here:

You: Hello.

Voice: Hello, may I ___________________

You: ___________________?

Voice: My name is ________________.

___________________ gave me your number.

You: Okay. So you are _________________

Voice: I need to know ________________________________________.

Should I come ______________________________________?

You: Why do you need my notes?

Voice: ______________________________________________.

You: Hmmmm. Come_____________________.

Voice: _______________________________

You: Bye.

Voice: Thank _____________________________

## 5. Complete this conversation between two friends

Salma: Hi __________________________?

Sujatha: Hi __________________________? It has been _______________________.

Salma: What ____________________________________?

Sujatha: I am in ______________________________. How about ________________?

Salma: I am a teacher in ____________________________.

Sujatha: Good. How is ______________________________?

Salma: Thank you for asking. They ________________________.

How is your_____________?

Sujatha: They are ___________________________.Sister is married now.

Salma: Nice to ______________________________.

Sujatha: Shall we have coffee ______________________________.

Salma: Yes.______________________________

Now think of a situation and write a conversation where two speakers have five turns each.

______________________________________________________________________

______________________________________________________________________

______________________________________________________________________

______________________________________________________________________

______________________________________________________________________

______________________________________________________________________

______________________________________________________________________

______________________________________________________________________

______________________________________________________________________

______________________________________________________________________



With this we come to the end of this book. I stress once again it is with regular practice that one can speak and write with confidence. Do not give up when the going becomes challenging. You may not have enough free time or you may be tired at the end of a busy day. Do not let all these realities become excuses in not reaching your goal- knowing and using good English.

All the effort does pay when you are understood and told that as a nurse you communicate well. The praise may come to you from patients or their families or from your superiors or you may hear about it through somebody. Or you may never be praised. But the feeling of achievement you get when you know you are speaking well is everything.

Have a happy time with the English language.

# Index

# Index